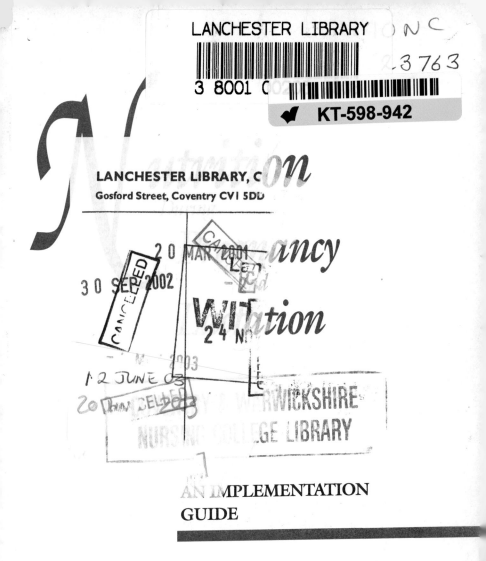

Nutrition During Pregnancy and Lactation

AN IMPLEMENTATION GUIDE

Subcommittee for a Clinical Application Guide
Committee on Nutritional Status During
    Pregnancy and Lactation
Food and Nutrition Board
Institute of Medicine
National Academy of Sciences

National Academy Press
Washington, D.C. 1992

National Academy Press • 2101 Constitution Avenue, NW • Washington, DC 20418

NOTICE: The project that is the subject of this report was approved by the Governing Board of the National Research Council, whose members are drawn from the councils of the National Academy of Sciences, the National Academy of Engineering, and the Institute of Medicine. The members of the committee responsible for the report were chosen for their special competences and with regard for appropriate balance.

This report has been reviewed by a group other than the authors according to procedures approved by a Report Review Committee consisting of members of the National Academy of Sciences, the National Academy of Engineering, and the Institute of Medicine.

The Institute of Medicine was chartered in 1970 by the National Academy of Sciences to enlist distinguished members of the appropriate professions in the examination of policy matters pertaining to the health of the public. In this, the Institute acts under both the Academy's 1863 congressional charter responsibility to be an adviser to the federal government and its own initiative in identifying issues of medical care, research, and education.

This study was supported by project no. MCJ 117018 from the Maternal and Child Health Program (Title V, Social Security Act), Health Resources and Services Administration, U.S. Department of Health and Human Services.

Library of Congress Cataloging-in-Publication Data

Institute of Medicine (U.S.). Subcommittee for a Clinical Application Guide.
  Nutrition during pregnancy and lactation : an implementation guide / Subcommittee for a Clinical Application Guide, Committee on Nutritional Status during Pregnancy and Lactation, Food and Nutrition Board, Institute of Medicine, National Academy of Sciences.
       p. cm.
  Includes bibliographical references and index.
  ISBN 0-309-04738-2
  1. Pregnancy--Nutritional aspects. 2. Lactation--Nutritional aspects. 3. Nutrition counseling. I. Title.
  [DNLM: 1. Lactation. 2. Nutrition--in pregancy. 3. Prenatal Care--standards. WQ 175 I595n]
  RG559.I56 1992
  618.2'4--dc20
  DNLM/DLC
  for Library of Congress   92-19175
                                                                        CIP

Printed in the United States of America

The serpent has been a symbol of long life, healing, and knowledge among almost all cultures and religions since the beginning of recorded history. The image adopted as a logotype by the Institute of Medicine is based on a relief carving from ancient Greece, now held by the Staatlichemuseen in Berlin.

SUBCOMMITTEE FOR A CLINICAL APPLICATION GUIDE

CHRISTINE OLSON (*Co-Chair*), Division of Nutritional Sciences, Cornell University, Ithaca, New York

JUDY WILSON (*Co-Chair*), District of Columbia WIC State Agency, Commission of Public Health, Department of Human Services, Washington, D.C.

BARBARA ABRAMS, Program in Public Health Nutrition, School of Public Health, University of California, Berkeley, California

IRENE ALTON, Health Start Inc., St. Paul, Minnesota

RONALD A. CHEZ, Department of Obstetrics and Gynecology, University of South Florida, Tampa, Florida

PETER DALLMAN, Department of Pediatrics, University of California, San Francisco, California

PATRICIA DOLAN MULLEN, Center for Health Promotion Research and Development, School of Public Health, Houston, Texas

LISA L. PAINE, School of Public Health, Boston University, Boston, Massachusetts

MINDY ANN SMITH, Department of Family Practice, University of Michigan, Ann Arbor, Michigan

RICHARD A. WINDSOR (until February 15, 1991), School of Public Health, University of Alabama, Birmingham, Alabama

Staff

CAROL WEST SUITOR, Study Director
YVONNE L. BRONNER, Research Associate (until June 30, 1991)
SHEILA MYLET, Research Associate
GERALDINE KENNEDO, Administrative Assistant

Preface

Nutritional care is viewed as an essential component of prenatal care, but many women receive little or no guidance regarding nutrition as part of the health care they receive during the preconception, prenatal, or postpartum periods. This guide is motivated by the need for all health care providers to put into action that which is agreed to be desirable—the inclusion of nutritional care in comprehensive health care.

This guide provides practical, easy-to-use information and tools for many kinds of care providers to use with patients of different economic, social, and cultural backgrounds. Some nutrition problems require the expertise and skills of a registered dietitian or a nutritionist; these are indicated in appropriate places in the guide along with questions other care providers should ask to help them to identify nutritional problems. We encourage all members of the health care team, especially nurses and physicians, to become more involved in providing nutritional care from preconception through the postpartum period.

The IOM reports *Nutrition During Pregnancy*[1] and *Nutrition During Lactation*[2] provide the basis for most of the content areas and principal recommendations covered in this guide. As in those IOM reports, the focus is primarily on healthy women.

Breastfeeding promotion and support activities in this guide merit special attention. Such activities have been strongly supported by the Surgeon General's workshops on breastfeeding and human lactation, the *Surgeon General's Report on Nutrition and Health,*[3] and *Healthy*

People 2000.[4] The special needs of the breastfeeding mother-infant pair make it appropriate to include information on breastfeeding and to ensure that practitioners provide nutritional care for lactating women. Only basic information is included here, since many authoritative books and other resources are available.

Well-targeted, basic nutritional care can make an important contribution to the health of women and their families. Yet the use of this guide is only one step in promoting optimal nutrition during pregnancy and lactation. Action is also needed at the policy level and in related areas of health care. To benefit from the suggestions contained in this guide, women must have access to health care. In addition, steps must be taken to make it more economically feasible to include dietitians and nutritionists in the delivery of care to pregnant and lactating women. Young people must arrive at the reproductive period in their lives literate in the basics of nutrition and health and valuing their health as an important personal resource. The subcommittee urges action in these areas to enhance and make more effective the recommendations contained in the guide.

Christine Olson
Co-Chair, Subcommittee for a Clinical Application Guide

Judy Wilson
Co-Chair, Subcommittee for a Clinical Application Guide

Roy M. Pitkin
Chair, Committee on Nutritional Status During Pregnancy and Lactation

Dedication

This guidebook is dedicated to Joel C. Kleinman, 1946–1991. We warmly remember his contributions to the IOM report *Nutrition During Pregnancy* and his commitment to improving maternal and child health in the United States.

Acknowledgments

This project was made possible by a grant from the Maternal and Child Health Bureau, Health Resources and Services Administration, U.S. Department of Health and Human Services. During the development of this guidebook, many people made important contributions by providing the subcommittee with resource materials or special written reports, sharing their views during workshops, or otherwise serving as resource persons. In addition, more than 40 practitioners and academicians from across the nation reviewed a draft and provided the basis for extensive revisions prior to formal review. The subcommittee thanks Louise Acheson, Case Western Reserve, Cleveland, Ohio; Joanna Asarian, WIC Program, Los Angeles, Calif.; Karen Bertram, Perinatal Unit, Sacramento, Calif.; Dan Bier, Wisconsin Association for Perinatal Care, Madison, Wisc.; Judith E. Brown, University of Minnesota, Minneapolis, Minn.; Doris Clements, Virginia Department of Health, Richmond, Va.; Annette Dickinson, Council for Responsible Nutrition, Washington, D.C.; Diane Dimperio, North Central Florida Maternal and Infant Care Project, Gainesville, Fla.; Ofelia Dirige, San Diego State University, San Diego, Calif.; Kittie Frantz, Santa Monica, Calif.; Phillip J. Goldstein, Sinai Hospital of Baltimore, Baltimore, Md.; Ann Gulbransen, Cleveland, Ohio; Terry F. Hatch, Carle Foundation Hospital, Urbana, Ill.; Barbara Heiser, Ellicott City, Md.; Eric Henley, Public Health Service Indian Hospital, Albuquerque, N.Mex.; Carol A. Hickey, University of Alabama, Birmingham, Ala.; Patricia Higgins, Albuquerque, N.Mex.; Vergie Hughes, Georgetown University Hospital, Washington, D.C.; Mary Ann Hylander, Takoma Park, Md.; Mildred Kaufman, Jacksonville, Fla.; John H. Kennell, Rainbow Baby Children's Hospital, Cleveland, Ohio; Karen Knoll, Minneapolis Department of Health, Minneapolis, Minn.; Mary Koenen, Holy Family Birth Center, Weslaco, Tex.; Ruth Lawrence, University of Rochester, Rochester, N.Y.; Minda Lazarov, Tennessee Department of Health, Nashville, Tenn.; Janet Lebeuf, North Carolina WIC Program, Raleigh, N.C.; Diana Lee, Department of Health Services, Emeryville, Calif.; R. Dee Legako, Edmond, Okla.; Barbara Luke, Johns Hopkins Hospital, Baltimore, Md.; Alice Lockett, District of Columbia General Hospital, Washington, D.C.; Stanley Malnar, Spokane, Wash.; Irwin R. Merkatz, Albert Einstein College of Medicine, Bronx, N.Y.; Sister Angela Murdaugh, Holy Family Birth Center, Weslaco, Tex.; Audrey Naylor, Wellstart, San Diego, Calif.; Vicky Newman, Wellstart, San Diego, Calif.; H. James Nickerson,

Marshfield Clinic, Marshfield, Wisc.; Donna O'Hare, Maternal and Infant Care-Family Planning Program, New York, N.Y.; Henry Osborne, WRC-TV, Washington, D.C.; Ruth Palombo, Department of Public Health, Boston, Mass.; Suzanne Pelican, Indian Health Service, Santa Fe, N.Mex.; Duc Quan, WIC Program, Anaheim Hill, Calif.; David Rath, Arkansas Department of Health, Little Rock, Ark.; Roger B. Rodrique, Wilmington, Del.; Eunice Romero-Gwynn, University of California, Davis, Calif.; Marjorie Scharf, Maternal and Infant Health, Philadelphia, Pa.; Christine A. Shannon, New Hampshire Division of Public Health Services, Concord, N.H.; Carolyn Sharbaugh, National Center for Education in Maternal and Child Health, Washington, D.C.; Mary Story, University of Minnesota Health Center, Minneapolis, Minn.; Peter C. Van Dyck, Utah Department of Health, Salt Lake City, Utah; Janet L. Washington, Brigham and Women's Hospital, Boston, Mass.; Doris Weyl-Feyling, University of California Medical Hospital, San Francisco, Calif.; Catherine Wong, San Francisco Department of Public Health, San Francisco, Calif.; Bonnie Worthington-Roberts, University of Washington, Seattle, Wash.; Michal Young, D.C. General Hospital, Washington, D.C.; and others who worked behind the scenes.

Feasibility testing of the guidebook occurred at 10 sites across the United States and led to further revisions. The subcommittee gives special thanks to the liaisons and participants at those sites, some of whom are listed here: Kenneth Berneis, Otsego, Mich.; Patty Brown, Mary Imogene Bassett Hospital, Cooperstown, N.Y.; Harriet Charney, Kaiser Permanente Medical Center, Hayward, Calif; Alfredo Czerwinski and Mary Lind, Kelsey Seybold Clinic, P.A., Houston, Tex.; Kim Deltano, St. Margaret's Hospital for Women, Boston, Mass.; Pat Franz, Model Cities Health Center, St. Paul, Minn.; Cecelia M. Jevitt, Tampa General Hospital, Tampa, Fla.; John Niles, Washington, D.C.; Susan Velasquez, Public Health Service Indian Hospital, Fort Defiance, Ariz.; Joe Weick, Oregon Health Sciences University, Portland, Or.

The subcommittee also expresses its appreciation to the staff at the Institute of Medicine who helped to guide this project to completion. In particular, we thank Carol W. Suitor, Study Director, for her outstanding support. Thanks also go to Catherine E. Woteki, Director of the Food and Nutrition Board; Gerri Kennedo, Administrative Assistant; Yvonne Bronner and Sheila Mylet, Research Associates; and Enriqueta C. Bond, Executive Officer of the IOM—and to consultants Betsy Turvene and Michael Hayes. In addition, staff at National Academy Press—especially Linda Humphrey and Sally Stanfield—were exceptionally helpful in the development and production of user-friendly versions of the guidebook.

Contents

I New Tools and Clinical Care Outlines

1

Introduction

Why Use This Guidebook?

- To help you deliver high quality nutritional care as a part of comprehensive health care for women before, during, and after pregnancy.

What Does the Guidebook Contain?

- a sample nutrition questionnaire to identify women who may be at nutritional risk;
- weight gain charts for pregnant women;
- a chart of prenatal weight gain recommendations;
- a body mass index (BMI) chart;
- a table of cutoff values for anemia, with adjustments for cigarette smoking and altitude;
- a chart of indications for vitamin/mineral supplementation;
- clinical care outlines that equip the practitioner with items to check on, tips, and practical information by type of visit; and
- supplementary information for delivering effective care.

Who Should Use This Guidebook?

- Primary care providers who care for women in the preconceptional, prenatal, or postpartum periods—obstetricians, family practice physicians, pediatricians, midwives, nurse-practitioners, nurses, physicians' assistants, dietitians, and others.
- Those involved in the education or training of the practitioners mentioned above.

Some of the care activities outlined here are carried out mainly by physicians or nurse-midwives. Other care providers refer to the medical record for related information.

Ways to Use This Book

- Look in Tab 1 to find forms and charts to assist with basic nutritional assessment.
- Look in Tabs 2–5 to find current recommendations for basic nutritional care before, during, and after pregnancy. The **bold italics** identify sample questions and statements, and the "Explanatory Information" gives the rationale. Use the checklists at the beginning of these tabs as a ready reference.
- Read through Part II (Tabs 6–10) for useful background information.

Tips for Using This Book

Skim the book to spark ideas for improving nutritional care and to locate sections of special interest. Apply durable tape to the first tab in each section to make the tabs easier to use. Consider using the entire book as a step-by-step guide for integrating nutrition into health care.

Approach

This guidebook encourages health care providers to build on the woman's strengths and reinforce the positive aspects of her diet while working to change behaviors that increase health risks for either the woman or her baby. Regardless of the setting, the aim is for health care or its providers to have the following characteristics:

- care structured for easy access and continuity;
- providers familiar with the cultural backgrounds and social circumstances of the patients they serve;
- providers aware that their own culture influences their attitudes toward patients and the delivery of services;

- recommendations that consider the individual woman's needs, preferences, culture, and resources;
- interactions that convey respect and concern for the woman; and
- joint goal setting by the health care provider or team and the woman.

Terminology

In this guidebook, the term *dietitian* is used to represent a qualified nutrition professional, ordinarily a registered or a licensed dietitian or a nutritionist who is eligible for registration.

Dietitian Referral and Consultation

Enhanced nutrition services can be provided if the health care team includes a dietitian. In those instances in which a dietitian is not a member of the team, the subcommittee urges practitioners to make arrangements for outside referral to a dietitian if the woman needs specialized nutritional care. When such referral is impossible, consultation by the primary care provider with a dietitian is indicated. For more information on this, see the companion document *Nutrition Services in Perinatal Care*,[5] which outlines the personnel requirements and the knowledge and skills needed to deliver nutrition services of varying degrees of complexity.

Record Keeping

Record keeping is a vital aspect of nutritional care delivery that is not covered explicitly in this guidebook. It varies depending on the type of record keeping system used and conventions at the health care facility.[6] For example, the Popras III Form 1B (see POPRAS Ltd.[7]) includes easily identified places for recording most of the prenatal nutrition-related information, and the Hollister Prenatal Module includes similar items.[8] The American

College of Obstetricians and Gynecologists antenatal record[9] does not include specific items for recording some of the information, but the nonspecific items ("Other") could be used for documentation.

Introduction to the Nutrition Questionnaire

This nutrition questionnaire is intended to serve as an example of a useful tool that many women can complete on their own before meeting with the provider. Adaptations would be needed for many clinical settings. For example, it may be necessary to substitute the names of foods and beverages commonly consumed by a specific ethnic group. The questions are intended to be easy for women to answer even if they do not read or write very well. If a face-to-face interview is necessary because the woman cannot read, it is desirable to rephrase the questions to make them open-ended. For example, Question 2 "Do you skip meals at least 3 times a week?" becomes "How often do you skip meals?" and Question 5 becomes "What foods do you avoid for health or religious reasons?"

Although food intake on the previous day is often typical of usual intake, certain life events may make it atypical. This must be assessed (as in Question 13) and considered in interpreting yesterday's reported intake. Nonetheless, the foods circled on the questionnaire provide a useful starting point for identifying possible areas of dietary concern and the need for further face-to-face questioning.

The questionnaire is not meant to replace more extensive ones used in many practices. It is recommended primarily for practices that have not yet included a nutrition questionnaire as a part of routine health care. Guidelines for choosing more extensive approaches to dietary assessment are included in Tab 7, pages 97 to 100.

Nutrition Questionnaire

What you eat and some of the life-style choices you make can affect your nutrition and health now and in the future. Your nutrition can also have an important effect on your baby's health. Please answer these questions by circling the answers that apply to you.

Eating Behavior

1. Are you frequently bothered by any of the following? (circle all that apply):

Nausea   Vomiting   Heartburn   Constipation

2. Do you skip meals at least 3 times a week?   No   Yes

3. Do you try to limit the amount or kind of food you eat to control your weight?   No   Yes

4. Are you on a special diet now?   No   Yes

5. Do you avoid any foods for health or religious reasons?   No   Yes

Food Resources

6. Do you have a working stove?   No   Yes
Do you have a working refrigerator?   No   Yes

7. Do you sometimes run out of food before you are able to buy more?   No   Yes

8. Can you afford to eat the way you should?   No   Yes

9. Are you receiving any food assistance now?   No   Yes
(circle all that apply):

Food stamps   School breakfast   School lunch
WIC   Donated food/commodities   CSFP
Food from a food pantry, soup kitchen, or food bank

10. Do you feel you need help in obtaining food?   No   Yes

Food and Drink

11. Which of these did you drink yesterday? (circle all that apply):

Soft drinks   Coffee   Tea   Fruit drink
Orange juice   Grapefruit juice   Other juices   Milk
Kool-Aid®   Beer   Wine   Alcoholic drinks
Water   Other beverages (list) _____

12. Which of these foods did you eat yesterday?
(circle all that apply):

Cheese   Pizza   Macaroni and cheese
Yogurt   Cereal with milk
Other foods made with cheese (such as tacos,
enchiladas, lasagna, cheeseburgers)

Corn	Potatoes	Sweet potatoes	Green salad
Carrots	Collard greens	Spinach	Turnip greens
Broccoli	Green beans	Green peas	Other vegetables

Apples	Bananas	Berries	Grapefruit
Melon	Oranges	Peaches	Other fruit

Meat	Fish	Chicken	Eggs
Peanut butter	Nuts	Seeds	Dried beans

Cold cuts	Hot dog	Bacon	Sausage
Cake	Cookies	Doughnut	Pastry
Chips	French fries		

Other deep-fried foods, such as fried chicken or egg rolls

Bread	Rolls	Rice	Cereal
Noodles	Spaghetti	Tortillas	

Were any of these whole grain?   No   Yes

13. Is the way you ate yesterday the way you
usually eat?   No   Yes

Life-Style

14. Do you exercise for at least 30 minutes on
a regular basis (3 times a week or more)?   No   Yes

15. Do you ever smoke cigarettes or use
smokeless tobacco?   No   Yes

16. Do you ever drink beer, wine, liquor, or any
other alcoholic beverages?   No   Yes

17. Which of these do you take?
(circle all that apply):

Prescribed drugs or medications

Any over-the-counter products (such as aspirin, Tylenol®,
antacids, or vitamins)

Street drugs (such as marijuana, speed, downers, crack, or
heroin)

Interpretation of Nutrition Questionnaire

When looking over the woman's responses to the nutrition questionnaire, look at the items below for reasons for concern, sources of additional information, and suggested follow-up questions or actions. The numbers below match the question numbers.

Introduce the follow-up questions by telling the woman that: **It would help us with planning your care if you would answer some additional questions.**

Eating Behavior

1. Regardless of the responses on the questionnaire, ask: **How has your appetite been recently?**

At the initial prenatal visit, ask:

- **Is _____ [symptom] keeping you from eating or from drinking liquids?**
- **What have you done to try to decrease _____ [these symptoms]? Has this helped?**

Strategies for managing nausea and vomiting are on page 47; those for heartburn and constipation are on page 63.

2. Skipping meals one or more times daily, three or more times per week, may lead to inadequate nutrient intake or to the eating of large meals, which may cause discomfort.

3. If yes, ask, **Do you sometimes feel that you can't stop eating?** Women who consistently restrict their food intake to control weight may have difficulty changing to more appropriate eating habits to support a healthy pregnancy or may find they gain large amounts of weight when their eating becomes less restricted. Further assessment may be desirable.

4. If on a special diet, ask, **What kind? Who told you to follow this diet?** Women who require special diets benefit from referral to a dietitian. Self-imposed diets require further assessment.

5. If yes, ask, *What foods do you avoid?* Women who avoid major sources of nutrients may benefit from diet counseling or from vitamin/mineral supplementation or both. See supplement chart, page 17.

Food Resources

6–10. A "Yes" answer to Questions 7 or 10, or a "No" answer to Question 8 indicates the probable need to facilitate linkage with food assistance programs, income support programs, or both, especially if the woman is not receiving appropriate benefits. (See responses to Question 9 and check the medical record for information about public assistance, Medicaid, and unemployment insurance.) See Tab 10, pages 114–115, for information about food and nutrition programs.

Food and Drink

11. Soft drinks, coffee, tea, fruit drink, Kool-Aid®, and alcoholic beverages provide few essential nutrients and often crowd out better sources of nutrients. Milk is the only dependable food source of vitamin D. Orange juice is an important source of vitamin C and folate. Drinking of alcoholic beverages is not recommended for pregnant women or for women trying to conceive. Drinking of two to three servings of caffeinated beverages is unlikely to have adverse effects.

12. Foods that contain milk, cheese, or yogurt are all good sources of calcium, as well as many other minerals, protein, and vitamins. Many are also good sources of vitamin A. A calcium supplement is recommended for women who do not drink milk or do not eat one of these foods daily.

The vegetables listed are mainly those most commonly eaten across the United States. Carrots, spinach and other greens, sweet potatoes, and winter squash are very high in vitamin A. Asparagus, broccoli, avocados, okra, brussels sprouts, greens, and corn provide more folate per usual serving than do other vegetables. If no vegetables other than potatoes or corn are eaten regularly, dietary guidance and vitamin/mineral supplementation may be appropriate.

The fruits listed are mainly those most commonly eaten across the United States. Citrus fruits and juices, strawberries, and cantaloupe are especially good sources of vitamin C and folate. If no juices or fruits are eaten regularly, dietary guidance and vitamin/mineral supplementation may be appropriate.

Meat, poultry, fish, eggs, and beans provide protein, iron, zinc, many other minerals, and vitamins.

Cold cuts, pastries, and deep-fried foods are all high in fat and calories. Frequent use of high-fat foods may crowd out better sources of nutrients.

Grains provide vitamins, minerals, protein, and energy without providing much fat. Whole grains are a source of fiber. Highly fortified cereals such as Total® and Special K® provide vitamins in amounts comparable to those in standard-strength vitamin pills.

See pages 27, 28, and 45 for information about dietary guidance.

13. If intake was not usual, ask: **What was different about the way you ate yesterday?** If a problem with diet is suspected, it is desirable to assess intake more thoroughly. (See Tab 7.)

Life-Style

14. Pregnant women need guidance concerning safe activity levels and may need encouragement to continue moderate excercise.

15–17. A "Yes" answer (indicating that the woman ever uses tobacco, alcoholic beverages, or street drugs) calls for questions to determine if any changes in behavior have been made already:

- *About how much did you use this past week?*
- *Is this more or less than before?*
- *Do you want to stop?*

16. For women who ever drink alcoholic beverages, ask the next four questions.

> *a. How many drinks does it take to make you feel high?*
> *b. Have people annoyed you by criticizing your drinking?*
> *c. Have you felt you ought to cut down on your drinking?*
> *d. Have you ever had a drink first thing in the morning to steady your nerves or get rid of a hangover?*

A response to Question 16*a* of more than two drinks indicates tolerance to alcohol and is given 2 points. Score 1 point for each additional "Yes" answer. A score of 2 or more indicates an at-risk drinker.[10]

17. See follow-up material under Tab 2, pages 25 and 26, or Tab 3, page 42.

Charts for Assessing Weight

Body Mass Index

Use the chart on page 14 to estimate the woman's prepregnancy body mass index (BMI) category. Find the number that is closest to her height (inches are at the bottom margin, centimeters at the top). Then find the number closest to her weight (pounds are on the left, kilograms on the right). Now, find the point where the height and weight intersect. For example, a woman who is 65 inches tall and weighed 145 lb had a normal prepregnancy BMI—slightly higher than 24.

The chart below also gives the weight classifications and BMI ranges.[1]

Relative Weight Classification	Prepregnant BMI
Underweight	<19.8
Normal	19.8–26.0
Overweight	26.1–29.0
Obese	>29.0

Weight Gain During Pregnancy

Plot the pregnant woman's weight on the weight gain chart using one of the following methods. Use a colored pen to highlight the dashed line that corresponds to the woman's BMI category.

When prepregnancy weight is known: (1) write the woman's prepregnancy weight, rounded to the nearest pound, on the blank line to the left of the zero on the left-hand side of the grid; then mark an x at 0 gain for 0 weeks; (2) fill in the rest of the blanks along the left side of the grid, adding the prepregnancy weight to the weight gain shown at each horizontal line (for example, if the woman's prepregnancy weight was 121 lb, 126 lb is the prepregnancy weight plus a 5-lb gain, 131 lb is the prepregnancy weight plus a 10-lb gain, and so on); (3) at each subsequent visit, have the woman plot her current weight at the point corresponding to the number of weeks of gestation.

If prepregnancy weight is not known: (1) mark an x on the highlighted dashed line at the point that corresponds to the correct number of weeks of gestation; (2) move horizontally from that point to find the corresponding point on the vertical axis, which shows weight, and write the woman's current weight to the left of that point; (3) if the woman's initial weight does not fall on a horizontal line, estimate the number to write in the blank at the nearest horizontal line (add or subtract up to 2 lb); then fill in the rest of the blanks up the left side of the grid by adding 5 lb for each horizontal line.

Chart for Estimating Body Mass Index (BMI) Category and BMI

Directions

To find BMI category (e.g., obese), find the point where the woman's height and weight intersect. To estimate BMI, read the bold number on the dashed line that is closest to this point.

Height, cm

Weight, kg

Weight, lb

Height, in

Obese · High · Normal · Low

Prenatal Weight Gain Chart

Prepregnancy BMI <19.8 (·······), Prepregnancy BMI 19.8–26.0 (Normal Body Weight) (- - - - -), Prepregnancy BMI >26.0 (— — —)

Date	Weeks of Gestation	Weight	Notes

Name

Date of Birth

E.D.C.

Height

Prepregnant Weight

Weight and Weight Gain, lb

Weeks of Pregnancy

Adapted from *Nutrition During Pregnancy*.[1]

Laboratory Tests and Nutrient Supplements

The selection of supplements depends on the presence of anemia, as determined by analysis of hemoglobin or hematocrit, and the presence of risk factors, as determined by a history that includes diet and by physical examination. Begin routine iron supplementation for all pregnant women by the 12th week of gestation.

The taking of vitamin/mineral supplements does not lessen the need for the consumption of a nutritionally balanced diet, nor should it be used to replace nutrition education and counseling. Women should be cautioned about taking self-prescribed vitamins, minerals, or other supplements because of the potential of such supplements for producing nutrient imbalances, excesses, or toxicities.

TABLE 1. Cutoff Values for Anemia for Women[a]

Pregnancy Status	Hemoglobin (g/dl)	Hematocrit (%)
Nonpregnant	12.0	36
Pregnant		
Trimester 1	11.0	33
Trimester 2	10.5	32
Trimester 3	11.0	33

[a]From CDC.[11] See Tab 9, Table 3, for corrections for high altitude.

TABLE 2. Cutoff Values for Anemia for Women Who Smoke Cigarettes[a,b]

Cigarettes per day	10-20		21-40	
Pregnancy Status	Hct[c] (g/dl)	Hgb[d] (%)	Hct (g/dl)	Hgb (%)
Nonpregnant	12.3	37	12.5	37.5
Pregnant				
Trimester 1	11.3	34	11.5	34.5
Trimester 2	10.8	33	11.0	33.5
Trimester 3	11.3	34	11.5	34.5

[a]From CDC.[11]
[b]No adjustment is necessary for women who smoke less than 10 cigarettes daily.
[c]Hgb = hemoglobin.
[d]Hct = hematocrit.

Indications for Nutrient Supplementation

Reproductive Period and Condition	Low-Dose (30 mg) Iron[a,b]	60–120 mg of Iron[b,c]	Low-Dose Multivitamin/ Mineral Preparation[d]	600 mg of Calcium
Preconception, interconception				
Iron deficiency anemia		✓	✓	
Pregnancy				
Normal	✓			
Complete vegetarian			✓	
Multiple gestation			✓	
Poor-quality diet and resistant to change			✓	
Heavy cigarette smoking			✓	
Alcohol abuse			✓	
Under age 25, consuming no calcium-rich milk products, and resistant to change			✓[e]	✓
Iron deficiency anemia		✓	✓	
Lactation				
Low energy intake			✓[e]	
Low intake of milk products			✓[e]	✓
Iron deficiency anemia		✓	✓	

[a]Begin routine iron supplementation for all pregnant women by the 12th week of gestation.
[b]Iron should be taken with juice or water, apart from meals.
[c]Therapeutic doses of iron should be taken apart from other supplements.
[d]For the suggested composition, see Tab 9.
[e]The vitamin supplement is indicated to supply vitamin D. Regular exposure to sunshine reduces the need for this supplement.

2

The Preconception/ Interconception Visit

Checklist

Gathering Information

Questions

☐ Administer nutrition questionnaire and check medical records to determine factors that may affect nutritional status and needs

☐ Indications of an eating disorder?

☐ Pregnancy planned?

Physical Examination

☐ General appearance

☐ Weight and height: determine body mass index category

☐ Anemia: Hemoglobin <12.0 g/dl (nonsmokers)

Basic Guidance

☐ The Dietary Guidelines

☐ Physical activity

☐ Weight maintenance or normalization

☐ Avoidance or cutting back on the use of harmful substances

Addressing Problems

- ☐ Assist with access to food
- ☐ Treat disorders requiring diet therapy
- ☐ Treat anemia: For iron deficiency anemia—60 to 120 mg of elemental iron daily; at a different time of day, give 15 mg of zinc and 2 mg of copper as part of a vitamin/mineral supplement
- ☐ Consider folate supplementation to help prevent recurrent neural tube defects
- ☐ Combat the use of harmful substances

The Preconception/ Interconception Visit

The preconception/interconception visit may be conducted when a woman of childbearing potential has a routine health care visit. The major goals of nutrition-related care are to identify women who are at nutritional risk and to provide appropriate nutrition management.

For women who are actively preparing for pregnancy and want additional information, see Tab 3, "The First Prenatal Visit."

It is assumed that before meeting with the health care provider the woman will complete a nutrition questionnaire. If the woman has difficulty reading or other special circumstances apply, the questions should be asked in person in the woman's native language, using an approach that encourages unguided responses.

Gathering Information

Check the medical record and the nutrition questionnaire to identify relevant questions and avoid unnecessary repetition. Useful sociodemographic data includes maternal age, ethnic background, marital status, and evidence of low income.

History—Sample Questions

Sociodemographic, Obstetric, Medical, and Life-Style Factors

- *What vitamins, minerals, or other supplements are you taking? How much? How often? Why?*
- *Have you had anemia, "low blood," or "low iron"?*
- *Are you breastfeeding now?*
- *Are you planning to become pregnant in the next year?*

Weight Status

- *How do you feel about your current weight?*
- *Have you ever been underweight? Overweight? What, if anything, did you do about it?*
- If an eating disorder is suspected, ask: *Does it bother you to know that you are going to be weighed?* If yes, *When you know you will be weighed, do you ever eat less? Force yourself to vomit? Use laxatives or diuretics? Exercise a lot?*
- *Have you recently gained or lost weight? How much? How fast? Were you trying to lose weight?* If yes, *Using what type of plan?*

Dietary Practices

See Questions 2 through 5 and 11 through 13 on the nutrition questionnaire.

Use of Harmful Substances

See Questions 15 through 17 on the nutrition questionnaire.

Physical Examination

General Appearance

Check for healthy gums, teeth, throat, and skin; overall physique; and amount and distribution of body fat. Observe the woman for signs of depression, poverty, battering, and poor hygiene.

Weight-for-Height Status

(Tab 1 contains recommended tools.)

- Measure height without shoes.
- Measure weight.
- Determine relative weight for height using body mass index (BMI) (see BMI chart in Tab 1).

Laboratory Evaluation

- Determine the hemoglobin or hematocrit value. If applicable, correct the value for smoking (Tab 1, page 16) or altitude (Tab 9, page 110) or both.
- Perform additional tests if appropriate. According to the history and physical examination, it may be advisable to do a lipid screen, a glucose screen, or other indicated blood or urine analyses.

Explanations

History

Sociodemographic, Obstetric, Medical, and Life-Style Factors

Nondietary factors may influence a woman's nutrient requirements, affect her ability to achieve adequate nutrition, signal previous problems with nutrition during pregnancy or lactation, or indicate the need for special approaches to care.

Excessive use of vitamin and mineral supplements is to be avoided. Vitamin A at high levels is a documented teratogen, and women considering pregnancy should be encouraged to discontinue vitamin A supplements, especially at dosages exceeding 800 RE (~4,000 IU) daily. Supplemental folate taken periconceptionally appears to help prevent neural tube defects in women who have previously had an affected pregnancy.[12] Preventing or resolving anemia is encouraged as part of general health promotion. A currently breastfeeding woman who is considering becoming pregnant has increased nutritional requirements. A woman who is planning a pregnancy can be given specific health and nutrition guidelines.

Weight Status

A woman's perceptions of her weight status may influence her nutrition now as well as during pregnancy. Rapid, substantial weight loss may decrease a woman's ability to conceive, as may obesity. Preoccupation with weight, widely fluctuating weight, or excessive exercise or dieting signals the need to assess the woman for a potential eating disorder.

Dietary Practices

Women who have poor appetites, who skip meals often, or who are purposely limiting their food intake may eat too little food to support a moderate body weight. Women on special diets for medical conditions may need assistance from a dietitian to modify food intake in support of their own health and a healthy pregnancy. Women who omit a major food group from their diets may have inadequate intakes of nutrients supplied by that food group.

Use of Harmful Substances

The use of cigarettes, smokeless tobacco, alcoholic beverages, or illegal drugs is a health risk for women regardless of whether they are pregnant. Furthermore, it may adversely affect nutrition. (See box on the next page.)

See "Information About Drugs," Tab 10, for sources of information about prescription medications and over-the-counter products.

Physical Examination

General Appearance

Signs of an eating disorder include dental enamel erosion, little subcutaneous fat, and (rarely) swollen parotid glands and callouses on the knuckles. Untreated dental disease, depression, battering, and other problems may interfere with adequate nutrient intake. Poor hygiene may be suggestive of life circumstances that interfere with adequate nutrient intake.

Weight-for-Height Status

Obesity increases the risk of developing many chronic diseases and complications of pregnancy. Low weight for height increases the risk of delivering a low birth weight baby.

Laboratory Evaluation

A positive screen for anemia (hemoglobin <12.0 g/dl, nonsmokers), elevated blood lipids, or other abnormal conditions call for additional testing or intervention.

Basic Guidance

General

- Affirm something positive, such as: ***I'm glad to see that you exercise regularly. It's a good habit with many health benefits.***
- Encourage healthful eating practices and exercise to achieve or maintain a healthy weight (BMI within the normal range shown on page 13).
- Using appropriate materials, provide guidance on sound eating practices based primarily on the Dietary Guidelines and indicate that these practices also help prevent chronic diseases such as cancer and heart disease.

Basic Dietary Guidance

There are numerous ways to achieve desirable dietary intakes of nutrients and of other beneficial food components such as fiber. An appropriate guide encourages the woman to aim for intakes such as those described in the Dietary Guidelines[13]: 2 servings of fruit; 3 of vegetables; 6 to 11 of grains; 2 of low-fat meat, fish, or poultry or of legumes; and 2 to 3 of low-fat, calcium-rich milk products such as low-fat milk, cheese, or yogurt. Vegetables can be grouped with fruits if desired, legumes can be counted as vegetables, and potatoes or viandas (starchy vegetables used by some Hispanics) can be substituted for grains. The actual number of servings suggested is of less importance than finding a guide to which the women can relate—one that includes practical and culturally acceptable suggestions for eating well. (To many people, one serving of rice or pasta would equal four servings of the size [$1/2$ cup] described in most nutrition education materials.)

Recommendations for All Women Based on Dietary Guidelines for Americans

- Eat a variety of foods.
- Choose a diet low in fat, saturated fat, and cholesterol. This reduces the risk of chronic disease and may help you manage your weight. Keeping fat intake under control also helps make room for foods that are rich in vitamins and minerals. Aim to have 2 servings daily of low-fat meat, fish, or poultry or of legumes. Also aim to have 2 to 3 servings of low-fat, calcium-rich milk products such as low-fat milk, cheese, or yogurt. One cup of milk or yogurt is an example of one serving.
- Choose a diet with plenty of vegetables, fruits, juices, and grain products. Choose whole-grain products at least part of the time. Aim to have 2 or more servings of fruit or juice, 3 or more servings of vegetables, and 6 to 11 servings of grains each day. One slice of bread and $^1/_2$ cup of rice, fruit, or vegetables are examples of one serving.
- Use sweets, sugars, and soft drinks only in moderation.
- Use salt and salty foods only in moderation. This helps prevent or control hypertension. However, restricted salt intake is not believed to be useful for the prevention or control of hypertension during pregnancy.

For the Woman:

Special Recommendations Before Pregnancy

- Maintain a healthy weight. Regular physical activity will help.
- If you need to gain or lose weight, do so gradually (no more than 1 to 2 lb/week).
- If you are trying to become pregnant and you ordinarily drink alcoholic beverages, omit alcohol or cut way back on the amount you drink.

Use of Medications, Supplements, and Harmful Substances

- Discourage the use of any kind of medication or supplement unless it is prescribed or approved by a physician who knows the woman is planning to become pregnant.
- Discourage the use of cigarettes, smokeless tobacco, alcoholic beverages, and illegal drugs.

Addressing Problems

Problems with Access to Food

- Provide assistance or refer the woman so that she can obtain assistance with food, housing, insurance, and income support programs. (See Tab 10 for information about federal food and nutrition assistance programs.)

Low Food or Nutrient Intake

- Help the woman develop a concrete plan for eating enough food to achieve or maintain a healthy weight. (See Tabs 7 and 8.)
- Engage her in identifying acceptable food sources of needed nutrients.
- Jointly decide on strategies for increasing nutrient intake from foods.

Disorders Requiring Diet Therapy

For women with common nutrition-related conditions (e.g., obesity, low body weight, or lactose intolerance), do one or more of the following:

- Provide individual or group counseling.
- Refer the woman to a dietitian.

If a woman has diabetes mellitus, phenylketonuria, renal disease, serious gastrointestinal disease, or other conditions requiring diet therapy, she should receive care from an experienced physician and dietitian. These providers should be consulted about appropriate follow-up care. (See "Referral to a Registered Dietitian," Tab 10.)

Women with eating disorders require comprehensive care by a specialized team.

Anemia

- If the hemoglobin is below 12.0 g/dl (nonsmokers), consider determining the serum ferritin. A low serum ferritin (<20 µg/liter)[14] indicates that the anemia is due to iron deficiency.
- For hemoglobin levels below 12.0 g/dl, start a therapeutic regimen of approximately 60 to 120 mg/day of ferrous iron, and give a multivitamin/mineral supplement that contains ~15 mg of zinc and ~2 mg of copper. See Tab 9.

- Consider other causes of anemia if it has not improved after 1 month.
- When the anemia has resolved, discontinue the high-dose iron. If a low dose of iron is needed because a chronic condition (such as heavy menstrual periods) originally caused the anemia, the iron can be provided with an iron-containing multivitamin/mineral preparation or the iron can be given alone.

Use of Harmful Substances

- Provide reinforcement for any constructive steps that have already been taken, provide assistance with quitting, and refer the woman for further evaluation or enrollment in an intensive treatment program as needed.
- If a pregnancy is planned, encourage the woman to view stopping or cutting down on substance use as a gift to her unborn child.
- Assist women in recovery to develop a sense of reasonable amounts of food to eat, especially if they are concerned about weight fluctuations.

History of Delivering an Infant with a Neural Tube Defect

The Centers for Disease Control recommends that if a woman has had a pregnancy involving a fetus or infant affected with a neural tube defect, she should consult her physician as soon as she plans a pregnancy. "Unless contraindicated, they should be advised to take 4 mg per day of folic acid starting at the time they plan to become pregnant. Women should take the supplement from at least 4 weeks before conception through the first 3 months of pregnancy. The dose should be taken only under a physician's supervision."[15] Folate supplementation after the third month of pregnancy does not protect against neural tube defects.

3

The First Prenatal Visit

Checklist

Use this checklist at the first prenatal visit if the woman has not had a recent preconceptional visit.

Gathering Information

Questions

☐ Administer questionnaire and review medical record
☐ Ask follow-up questions on eating behaviors, food use, discomforts, weight status
☐ Indications of an eating disorder?
☐ Infant feeding plans?

Physical Examination

☐ General appearance
☐ Breast examination
☐ Weight for height: estimate prepregnancy body mass index category if not charted—for use in giving weight gain advice
☐ Anemia: Hemoglobin <11.0 g/dl during first or third trimester, <10.5 g/dl during second trimester (non-smokers)
☐ Glucose screen (if first visit occurs after 24 weeks of gestation)

Basic Guidance

- [ ] Recommended diet for pregnancy
- [ ] Usual weight gain pattern and weight gain recommendations: normal prepregnancy weight, 25 to 35 lb; underweight, 28 to 40 lb; overweight, 15 to 25 lb; obese, at least 15 lb
- [ ] Iron supplementation (~30 mg/day) to begin by the 13th week of gestation to prevent anemia
- [ ] Appropriate physical activity, e.g., walking, swimming
- [ ] Avoidance of harmful substances
- [ ] Promotion of breastfeeding; support for the woman regardless of the feeding method chosen

Addressing Problems

At any stage of gestation

- [ ] Assist with access to food
- [ ] Treat disorders requiring diet therapy
- [ ] Treat anemia: For iron deficiency—60 to 120 mg of elemental iron daily; at a different time, 15 mg of zinc and 2 mg of copper given as part of a vitamin/mineral supplement
- [ ] Combat the use of harmful substances

First trimester

- [ ] Consider folate supplementation to help prevent recurrent neural tube defects
- [ ] Advise about control of nausea and vomiting associated with pregnancy

Second and third trimesters

- [ ] Counsel to improve diet (e.g., increasing dietary intake of calcium) and recommend nutrient supplements as needed—may be addressed earlier if control of nausea and vomiting associated with pregnancy is not a problem)
- [ ] Promote appropriate weight gain
- [ ] Advise about control of heartburn and constipation
- [ ] Help plan for eating well if on bed rest
- [ ] Treat inverted nipples (third trimester)

First Prenatal Visit
Modified Checklist

Use this checklist for a first-trimester visit following a recent pre-conception visit.

Gathering Information

Questions

☐ Review medical record
☐ Ask follow-up questions on eating behaviors, food use, previous recommendations
☐ Infant feeding plans?

Physical Examination

☐ General appearance
☐ Breast Examination
☐ Weight
☐ Anemia: Hemoglobin <11.0 g/dl (nonsmokers)

Basic Guidance

☐ Recommended diet for pregnancy
☐ Usual weight gain pattern and weight gain recommendations: normal prepregnancy weight, 25 to 35 lb; underweight, 28 to 40 lb; overweight, 15 to 25 lb; obese, at least 15 lb
☐ Iron supplementation (~30 mg/day) to begin by the 13th week of gestation
☐ Appropriate physical activity, e.g., walking, swimming
☐ Avoidance of harmful substances
☐ Promotion of breastfeeding; support for the woman regardless of feeding method chosen

Addressing Problems

☐ Identify continuing or new nutritional problems or concerns
  ☐ Controlling nausea and vomiting associated with pregnancy
  ☐ Access to food?

- [ ] Inadequate nutrient or energy intake related to food choices? Pica (the ingestion of nonfood substances)?
- [ ] Dietary control of chronic disorders?
- [ ] Anemia? For iron deficiency—60 to 120 mg of elemental iron daily; at a different time, 15 mg of zinc and 2 mg of copper and given as part of a vitamin/mineral supplement
- [ ] Continuation of folate supplementation to help prevent neural tube defects?
- [ ] Use of harmful substances?
- [ ] Set priorities
- [ ] Create a nutrition plan, focusing on concerns identified
- [ ] Arrange for referral for additional care as needed

The First Prenatal Visit

Ideally, the first prenatal visit will be a follow-up of the pre-conception/interconception visit. Since preconception visits are not yet common, however, this clinical care outline assumes that a preconception visit has not occurred.

The content of the first prenatal visit is influenced by the stage of gestation. For clarity, cross referencing is provided for topics that need to be addressed at specific times during pregnancy (e.g., guidance for controlling diet-related discomforts of pregnancy, testing for glucose tolerance).

It is assumed that before meeting with the health care provider the woman will complete a nutrition questionnaire. If the woman has difficulty reading or other special circumstances apply, the questions should be asked in person in the woman's native language, using an approach that invites unguided responses.

Information overload is to be avoided. By careful attention to information in the medical record, the nutrition questionnaire, the patient's responses to sample questions, and results of the physical examination and laboratory tests, the provider can set priorities and encourage active patient involvement in addressing those priorities.

The provider should consider the need to link the woman with support services, including those provided by case management and home visiting programs, especially when there is concern that this may be the only patient contact until delivery. Referral to WIC, when appropriate, is recommended as early in pregnancy as possible. (See "Referral to WIC," Tab 10, page 116.) If the first prenatal visit occurs shortly after a preconception visit, use the modified checklist as a guide.

Gathering Information

Check the medical record and the nutrition question-naire to identify relevant questions and avoid unnecessary repetition.

History—Sample Questions

Sociodemographic, Obstetric, Medical, and Life-Style Factors

- *What vitamins, minerals, or other supplements are you taking? How much? How often? Why?*
- *Have you had anemia, "low blood," or "low iron?"*
- *Are you currently breastfeeding?*

Weight

If height and recent weight are not available from the medical record, ask:

- *How much did you weigh at your last period?* If the woman is uncertain, ask: *Have you noticed a change in how well your clothes fit?*

Ask all pregnant women:

- *Have you ever been underweight? Overweight? What, if anything, did you do about it?*
- *How much weight do you think you should gain during this pregnancy?* If a low amount: *Does the thought of gaining at least __ lb bother you?*
- *How do you feel about your weight so far?*
- *What questions or concerns do you have about your weight or weight gain during pregnancy?*

Discomforts and Dietary Practices

See Questions 1 through 5 and 11 through 13 on the nutrition questionnaire.

Use of Harmful Substances

See "Interpretation of Nutrition Questionnaire," Questions 15 through 17.

Infant Feeding

- **What have you heard about breastfeeding?**
- **Have you ever breastfed?**
  If yes, ask: **How did it go?**
- **How do most of your friends feed their babies?**

Physical Examination

General Appearance

Check for healthy gums, teeth, throat, and skin; overall physique; and amount and distribution of body fat. Observe the woman for signs of depression, poverty, battering, and poor hygiene.

Breast Examination

Perform a breast examination to identify inverted nipples, breast surgery, cancer, or masses.

Weight and Weight-for-Height Status

- Accurately measure weight and height.
- Check medical record for recent preconceptional BMI. If unavailable, estimate it using the woman's height and recalled preconceptional weight and the BMI chart. (See Tab 1.)
- Determine weight-for-height category.

Laboratory Evaluation

- Determine the hemoglobin or hematocrit value. If applicable, correct the cutoff value for smoking (Tab 1, page 16) or altitude (Tab 9, page 110) or both.
- Perform additional tests if appropriate. According to the history, physical examination, and stage of gestation, it may be advisable to do a glucose screen or other indicated blood or urine analyses.

Explanations

History

Sociodemographic, Obstetric, Medical, and Life-Style Factors

Nondietary factors may influence a woman's nutrient requirements, affect her ability to achieve adequate nutrition, signal previous problems with nutrition during pregnancy or lactation, or indicate the need for special approaches to care.

Excessive use of vitamin and mineral supplements is to be avoided. Vitamin A at high levels is a documented teratogen, and pregnant women should avoid unprescribed supplements that contain vitamin A, especially at dosages exceeding 800 RE (~4,000 IU). Very early in pregnancy, supplemental folate may help prevent neural tube defects among women who have had a pregnancy affected by such a defect. Preventing or resolving anemia is encouraged as part of general health promotion. A pregnant woman who is currently breastfeeding has increased nutritional requirements.

Weight

Usual weight, weight change, and attitudes toward weight may influence the mother's pattern of weight gain during pregnancy.

Preoccupation with weight, widely fluctuating weight, or excessive exercise or dieting signals the need to assess for a potential eating disorder. Most women can alert the health care provider to large changes in weight even if they do not know their prepregnancy weight. Some women need special guidance to establish healthful weight gain goals for pregnancy. Because of their special concerns about body image, adolescents usually benefit from such guidance.

Discomforts and Dietary Practices

Women who have poor appetites, who skip meals often, or who are purposely limiting their food intake may eat too little food to support optimal weight gain and fetal growth during pregnancy. Women whose intake of food or fluids is minimal for a number of days because of lack of appetite, nausea, and/or vomiting may develop dehydration and ketosis. Usually, occasional nausea, vomiting, or loss of appetite is not a medical or nutritional concern. Almost all women will be free of gastrointestinal disease. However, an occasional woman will have a condition that requires active medical assessment and intervention. Women may need reassurance about their lack of ability to eat normally.

Women on special diets for medical conditions may need assistance from a dietitian to modify food intake in support of their own health and a healthy pregnancy. Women who omit a major food group from their diets may have inadequate intakes of nutrients supplied by that food group.

Use of Harmful Substances

Cigarette smoking is a major cause of low birth weight, other perinatal health problems, and many health problems unrelated to pregnancy and lactation. A safe lower limit for alcohol consumption during pregnancy is not known. Therefore, the only surely safe level of alcohol consumption for pregnant women is none. See box, page 26.

Infant Feeding

Breastfeeding is recommended for all infants in the United States under ordinary circumstances.[2] Many women make their infant feeding decisions before pregnancy or early in pregnancy—often without having contact with breastfeeding women or encouragement from health care providers.

Physical Examination

General Appearance

Signs of an eating disorder include dental enamel erosion, little subcutaneous fat, and (rarely) swollen parotid glands and calluses on the knuckles. Untreated dental disease, depression, battering, and other problems may interfere with adequate nutrient intake. Poor hygiene may be suggestive of life circumstances that interfere with adequate nutrient intake.

Breast Examination

Intervention for inverted nipples is recommended in the third trimester, but early in pregnancy women may need reassurance about their ability to breastfeed.

Weight and Weight-for-Height Status

The total amount of weight gain recommended for pregnant women depends largely on their BMI before pregnancy. (See the box on the next page.)

Laboratory Evaluation

Consider the nonsmoker anemic if her hemoglobin is below 11.0 g/dl in the first or third trimester or below 10.5 g/dl in the second trimester. A positive screen for anemia calls for iron therapy or additional testing. No other tests need to be done routinely solely to screen for nutritional problems.

Basic Guidance

General

- Affirm something positive, such as: ***By coming for prenatal care [or to this class], you are starting to take care of your baby.***
- Encourage healthful eating and weight gain.
- Encourage walking, swimming, dancing, or other appropriate exercise.

Dietary Practices

- Using appropriate materials, provide guidance on sound eating practices based primarily on the Dietary Guidelines. Use an approach that considers the woman's learning style, learning ability, literacy, native language, and other learner characteristics. People who do not organize eating by meals or food groups may benefit from dietary guidance that focuses mainly on foods, as in these examples:

Recommended Total Weight Gain Ranges for Pregnant Women[a,b]

Prepregnancy Weight-for-Height Category	Recommended Total Gain	
	lb	kg
Low (BMI <19.8)	28-40	12.5-18
Normal (BMI 19.8 to 26)	25-35	11.5-16
High (BMI >26.0 to 29.0)	15-25	7.0-11.5
Obese (BMI >29.0)	≥15	≥7.0

[a]Adapted from *Nutrition During Pregnancy*.[1]
[b]For singleton pregnancies. The range for women carrying twins is 35 to 45 lb (16 to 20 kg). Young adolescents (<2 years after menarche) and African-American women should strive for gains at the upper end of the range. Short women (<62 in. or <157 cm) should strive for gains at the lower end of the range.

- *Which of these snacks and fast foods do you like?* (Use the box in Tab 7.)
- *When would be a good time for you to eat a bowl of cereal with milk and fruit?*

• Assist with dietary improvement: reinforce positive aspects of the diet; help the woman to set realistic goals (e.g., one change at a time or small changes in related behaviors); and encourage her to commit to one change, possibly in writing (a contract for change).

- *What will you change? How much change is realistic right now?*
- *When will you do it? Where? How? Who might help you?*

• If the woman is currently breastfeeding and plans to continue, emphasize the importance of careful food selection and give concrete suggestions.

For the Pregnant Woman:

Special Dietary Recommendations for Pregnant Women

- Eat enough food to gain weight at the rate recommended by your health care provider, as shown on your weight gain chart. Include fruits, vegetables, grains, meat or meat alternates, and milk products in your meals and snacks every day.
- Eat small to moderate-sized meals at regular intervals, and eat nutritious snacks. This will help you to be comfortable and to have the best chance of getting all the nutrients you and your baby need.
- Take 3 or more servings of milk products daily, either with or between meals. One cup ($^{1}/_{2}$ pint) of milk is an example of one serving. Choose low-fat or skim milk products often.
- To absorb more iron, include some meat, poultry, fish, or vitamin-C-rich foods (such as orange juice, broccoli, or strawberries) in meals.
- Salt your food to taste unless your physician advises you to curb your salt intake because of a medical problem. Your need for salt increases somewhat during pregnancy.
- If you drink coffee or other caffeinated beverages such as cola, do so in moderation (2 to 3 servings or less daily).
- While you are pregnant, the only sure way to avoid the possible harmful effects of alcohol on the fetus is to avoid drinking alcoholic beverages entirely.

Weight

- Explain the weight gain recommendations for pregnancy shown in the box on page 44:
  - *Adequate* gain reduces the risk of low birth weight.
  - **Aim for a steady rate of weight gain:** weight gain in early pregnancy goes mainly toward the mother's tissues (such as placenta, amniotic fluid, uterus, expanded blood volume, energy reserves) to support the baby's growth; weight gain in later pregnancy goes mainly toward the growth of the baby. During the second and third trimesters, the recommended rate of gain is slightly more than 1 lb (0.5 kg) per week for women with low prepregnancy BMI, approximately 1 lb (0.5 kg) per week for women with moderate BMI, and $2/3$ lb (0.3 kg) per week for women with high BMI.
- Identify factors that may call for a higher weight gain during pregnancy (low prepregnancy weight-for-height status, young age [<2 years post menarche], African-American background, multiple gestation) or for weight gain at the lower end of the range (short maternal height).
- Use the appropriate weight gain chart to show the range and rate of weight gain recommended.
- Jointly agree upon a total weight gain goal, focusing on a range rather than a single number.
- Show the woman how to plot her prepregnancy weight (if it is available) and her current weight on the weight gain chart. Offer her a chart and help her start to use it. Suggest: **Please bring it with you next time.**
- Use the current measured weight as a baseline, and jointly set a realistic weight goal for the next visit.
- Explain that: **Weight can go up and down. Continue to eat well even if you think you're gaining weight too fast.**

> *For the Pregnant Woman:*
> ## Strategies for Managing Nausea and Vomiting
>
> - Keep crackers, melba toast, or dry cereal within reach of your bed. Eat some before getting up.
> - Eat frequent small meals.
> - Try to take adequate fluids even if you can't handle solids—for example, try clear juices and flat sugar-sweetened soft drinks.
> - Avoid drinking coffee and tea. Avoid drinking citrus fruit juices and water upon arising. Drink liquids mainly between meals.
> - Try to avoid cooking odors that make you feel ill.
> - Avoid or limit your intake of high-fat and spicy foods.

Comfort

- Provide anticipatory guidance for the woman's comfort. First trimester: control of nausea and vomiting, and early weight changes. Later in pregnancy: control of heartburn, constipation (see Tab 4).

Use of Supplements and Medications

- If not anemic: **Start taking a low-dose (~30 mg of elemental iron) iron supplement such as ferrous gluconate daily by** _____ (the thirteenth week of gestation).
- **Avoid using any kind of medication unless it is prescribed or approved by a physician who knows you are pregnant.**

Infant Feeding

- If interest is expressed in breastfeeding and there are no medical contraindications, support the choice. Offer educational materials, information about local classes, and a visit with a peer counselor.
- If bottle feeding is chosen, ask: **Have you considered breastfeeding? What have you heard about breastfeeding?** Offer written information on breastfeeding or alert the woman and her family to sources of visual and oral information, including breastfeeding counselors. Videotapes may be helpful.
- If the woman reports a history of breastfeeding problems or early discontinuation of breastfeeding, offer information that addresses these issues.
- For women with inverted nipples, reassure them by saying: **You have inverted nipples. We'll give you some extra help in the third trimester to make them ready for breastfeeding.** Document the treatment plan.

Addressing Problems

Problems with Access to Food

- Provide assistance or refer the woman so that she can obtain assistance with food, housing, insurance, and income support programs. (See Tab 10 for information about federal food and nutrition assistance programs and about referrals to WIC.)

Low Food or Nutrient Intake

- Help the woman develop a concrete plan for eating enough food to gain weight. (See Tabs 7 and 8.)
- Engage her in identifying acceptable food sources of needed nutrients. (For this purpose, try using

"Examples of Nutritious Snacks and Fast Foods" or "Ways to Increase Your Calcium Intake If You Avoid Most Milk Products" in Tab 7.)

- Jointly decide on strategies for increasing intake of nutrients from foods.
- Consider vitamin/mineral supplementation for women at risk of inadequate nutrient intake. For guidelines see the "Indications for Nutrient Supplementation" chart in Tab 1.

Disorders Requiring Diet Therapy

For women with common nutrition-related conditions (e.g., obesity, low body weight, lactose intolerance, or diet-related discomforts of pregnancy), do one or more of the following:

- Provide individual or group counseling.
- Refer the woman to the dietitian.

If a woman has diabetes mellitus, phenylketonuria, renal disease, serious gastrointestinal disease, or other conditions requiring diet therapy, she should receive care from an experienced physician and dietitian. These providers should be consulted about appropriate follow-up care. (See "Referral to a Registered Dietitian," Tab 10.)

Women with eating disorders require comprehensive care from a specialized team.

Anemia

- For hemoglobin levels below 11.0 g/dl in the first and third trimesters or below 10.5 g/dl in the second trimester (nonsmokers), start a therapeutic regimen of approximately 60 to 120 mg/day of ferrous iron. At a different time, give zinc and copper as part of a vitamin/mineral supplement. (See Tab 9.) Check hemoglobin level again in about 1 month.

Use of Harmful Substances

- Provide reinforcement for any constructive steps that have already been taken, provide assistance with quitting, and refer the woman to evaluation or treatment programs as needed.
- Encourage the woman to view stopping or cutting down on substance use as a gift to her unborn child.
- Assist women in recovery to develop a sense of reasonable amounts of food to eat, especially if they are concerned about high weight gain.

History of Delivering an Infant with a Neural Tube Defect

If the first prenatal visit occurs in the first trimester of pregnancy, the Centers for Disease Control recommends: "Unless contraindicated, they [women who have had a pregnancy involving a fetus or infant affected with a neural tube defect] should be advised to take 4 mg per day of folic acid . . . through the first 3 months of pregnancy. The dose should be taken only under a physician's supervision."[15] Folate supplementation after the third month of pregnancy does not protect against neural tube defects.

4
Follow-up Visits

Checklist

Gathering Information

Questions

☐ Behavior changes in response to nutrition-related advice or activities agreed upon during the last visit?

☐ Any additional problems or concerns related to food or supplement intake? Weight gain? Gastrointestinal symptoms? Health habits?

Physical Examination

☐ Weight; involve the woman in plotting her weight on chart; note weight change

☐ Anemia: repeat hemoglobin or hematocrit tests as needed for follow-up

☐ Glucose screen at 24 to 28 weeks of gestation

Basic Guidance

☐ Reinforce healthful practices

☐ Reinforce progress on specific behavior changes (e.g., increased intake of vegetables, eating breakfast, cutting back on cigarettes)

☐ Provide support for breastfeeding

Addressing Problems

☐ Identify continuing or new nutritional problems or concerns
   ☐ Discomforts of pregnancy?
   ☐ Anemia?
   ☐ Inadequate or excessive weight gain?
   ☐ Access to food?
   ☐ Dietary control of chronic disorders?
   ☐ Inadequate nutrient or energy intake related to food choices? Pica?
   ☐ Inverted nipples? (third trimester)
☐ Identify continuing or new obstetrical risk factors with implications for nutrition
   ☐ Multiple gestation?
   ☐ Need for bedrest?
   ☐ Gestational diabetes mellitus?
   ☐ Substance use?
   ☐ Need for vitamin/mineral supplements?
☐ Set priorities
☐ Create a nutrition plan, focusing on concerns identified
☐ Arrange for referral for additional care as needed

Follow-up Visits

These follow-up visits occur at intervals appropriate to the needs of the individual woman.

Follow-up visits allow the practitioner to monitor the progression of the pregnancy and determine priorities for nutritional care. Attention is directed toward problems such as low or excessive weight gain, inadequate nutrient intake, multiple gestation, gestational diabetes mellitus, anemia, inadequate resources, or gastrointestinal symptoms.

In this chapter, care that is appropriate at every visit is distinguished from care that is most relevant at specific times during the pregnancy.

4

Follow-up Visits

Gathering Information

Check the medical record and the nutrition questionnaire to identify relevant questions and avoid unnecessary repetition.

History—Sample Questions

General

If the nutrition questionnaire revealed problems at the time of the initial visit, consider administering it during the second and third trimesters as a quick way to identify continuing problems.

At *every* visit, interview the woman to determine behavioral changes made in response to recommendations at the previous visit (e.g., obtain feedback on referrals and specific changes in diet and substance use) and assess the woman's current status by inquiring about symptoms of nausea, vomiting, heartburn, constipation, and edema and her feelings about body image and weight gain.

Discomforts

- *Are you having a problem with nausea, vomiting, heartburn, constipation, or other discomforts?*
- If applicable, say: *I notice that you don't drink milk. Does drinking milk cause you any discomfort?* If yes, ask: *What kind? Have you tried drinking milk recently? How much milk does it take for you to get those symptoms?*
- *How do you feel about your weight so far?*

Dietary Practices

- If food intake is low or a major food group is avoided, ask: **Who shops for food in your household? Who plans the meals? Who cooks them? Do other family members complain if you fix something different from usual?**
- At an early prenatal visit, inquire about pica: **Some women eat things like clay, starch, or baking soda when they are pregnant. Do you eat any of these kinds of things? What? How much? How often?**
- Sample questions concerning the diet include:
  - **Has your appetite changed? How?**
  - **What special problems or concerns do you have about food or eating?**
  - **How much X are you eating now?**
  - **How are you using the milk that you get through WIC?**

Supplements

- **How often do you take your iron supplement? Do you take it with or without food? What liquid do you take with it?**
- **Have you noticed any changes in the way you feel since you started taking the iron? Tell me more about it.**
- If there are young children in the household, ask: **Where do you keep the pills?**

Behavioral Changes

- **What changes in exercise have you made?**
- **How much have you been walking?**
- If the woman had been smoking or using some other harmful substance, ask: **Have you tried to quit? To cut down? What have you done to stop X (behavior) since you were here last?**

- If the woman stopped for this pregnancy, ask:
  Have you been able to stay off?
- **How many cigarettes are you smoking now?**
- If specific strategies were suggested, ask questions such as:
  - **What did you think of the AA (or AlaTeen) meeting?**
  - **Did you attend the class on using WIC foods?**
  - **Did you pick up your WIC vouchers?**
  - **How often do you eat the cereal that WIC provides?**

Physical Examination

At every visit, obtain and record objective data:

- Weigh the woman or have her weigh herself.
- Plot her weight on the grid.
- Check the fundal height.
- Check for pretibial and facial edema.

Indications to assess weight gain further are shown in the box.

Weight Changes That Signal the Need for Further Evaluation in the Second and Third Trimesters

Women of at least moderate weight (Prepregnancy BMI >19.8):
- Gain of less than 2 lb (1 kg) in any single month

Obese women:
- Gain of less than 1 lb (0.5 kg) in any single month

All pregnant women
- Continuing pattern of less than recommended gain or of much higher than recommended weight gain
- Gain of more than 6.5 lb (3 kg) in any month

Laboratory Evaluation

- *Hemoglobin or Hematocrit.* Follow up on anemia in women in whom anemia is suspected or was previously diagnosed. For nonsmokers, hemoglobin should be ≥10.5 g/dl in the second trimester and ≥11.0 g/dl in the first and third trimesters.
- *Glucose screen:* A fasting 50-g, 1-hour post-glucose challenge test between 24 and 28 weeks of gestation is ordinarily recommended.

Explanations

History

Discomforts

Dietary measures can help relieve nausea (page 47), heartburn and constipation (page 63), and symptoms of lactose intolerance (such as abdominal cramps and explosive diarrhea that occur within an hour after drinking milk) (page 101). No well-conducted studies support special dietary measures for the treatment of leg cramps.

Dietary Practices

Strategies for dietary improvement may be strongly influenced by the availability of food, the degree of control the woman has over obtaining and preparing food, and her appetite.

Specific questions based on the recommendations made during the previous visit demonstrate a concern for the woman. The practice of pica (eating nonfood substances) may limit nutrient intake and have adverse hematologic or gastrointestinal effects.

Supplements

Many women need extra guidance to promote comfort, compliance, and safety when the use of vitamin/mineral supplements is indicated.

Behavioral Changes

Stopping substance use and improving diet quality are often difficult. Several encounters may be needed to achieve desirable change. Encouragement often helps women who have difficulty making appointments, accessing WIC, and making or maintaining behavioral changes. New problems may occur, which routine screening will help to identify. If desirable changes have occurred, the health professional's affirmation and reinforcement help to improve the woman's sense of self-esteem and promote healthful practices.

Physical Examination

A typical weight gain in the first trimester is 3 to 8 lb (~1 to 3.5 kg). Weight loss is often a sign of low food intake resulting from the nausea, vomiting, and poor appetite that are normal at this time. It could also be a sign of dehydration or of low intake associated with poor adjustment to pregnancy. Lack of weight gain is not ordinarily a major problem in the first trimester. A documented large weight gain during the first trimester may indicate the need for further assessment of dietary intake and physical activity, especially among overweight and obese women. Substantial weight gain by underweight women is usually desirable.

Adequate weight gain for BMI status suggests adequate energy intake but does not guarantee diet quality. The average weekly amount of weight gained increases in the second trimester, and women may express more concerns about their body image. High or low weight gain may result from measurement errors, dietary problems, edema, or other causes. A low weight gain combined with a low fundal height is of concern because of the possibility of fetal growth restriction.

Laboratory Evaluation

Resolving anemia may improve the mother's sense of well-being by relieving shortness of breath, fatigue, headache, and dizziness. Infants of iron-deficient mothers may have an increased risk of low birth weight, prematurity, and perinatal mortality. A positive glucose screen calls for diagnostic testing for glucose tolerance.

Basic Guidance

General

- Whenever possible, involve the partner and family or friends in activities to promote social support for improved nutrition and health.
- Positively reinforce healthful behaviors and progress toward any goals set at the previous visit.

Weight

- At every visit, involve the mother in plotting her weight on her weight gain chart and in interpreting her pattern of gain. Discuss implications. ***Do you have any more questions or concerns about your weight?***
- On the basis of the assessment, jointly set a new weight gain goal. Aim for the target rate of weight gain, even if it means exceeding the original goal.
- If this is a multiple gestation, revise weight gain recommendations to about 1.5 lb (0.75 kg) per week for twins, more for triplets.

Diet and the Avoidance of Harmful Substances

- At every visit, encourage a healthful diet, reinforce healthy dietary practices and the positive changes that have been made, encourage avoidance of potentially harmful substances, and address the woman's questions and concerns.
- As needed, try to involve the person responsible for food shopping and meal preparation when discussing strategies for improved dietary intake.

Promotion of Breastfeeding

Early in pregnancy, if there are no medical contraindications to breastfeeding:

- Provide information on the advantages and challenges of breastfeeding and bottle feeding.
- *X (name of person) would like to speak with you about her experience with breastfeeding. You can reach her by . . .*
- Support infant feeding decisions and encourage undecided women to breastfeed.
- As appropriate, provide anticipatory guidance on how to obtain assistance for successful lactation and realistic information about feeding frequency.

In the third trimester, resume the discussion of infant feeding. Include the partner in the discussion if possible.

- If breastfeeding is planned, build on previous experiences, address fears, explore possibilities for family support, and ask about work plans. If the woman's nipples are flat or inverted, consider breast shells and assist with their proper use. Provide education and encouragement.
- If bottle feeding is planned, address questions and concerns. Provide anticipatory guidance and support the mother.

- If the woman is uncertain about which feeding method to choose, ask what she and her partner see as the advantages and disadvantages of breastfeeding. Clarify misconceptions, provide information (using role models and audiovisuals), and encourage the woman to try breastfeeding at least for a short time.

Addressing Problems

Low Intake of Fluids and Foods

- Reassure the woman that occasional nausea and vomiting will not hurt the baby.
- Suggest strategies for relieving or avoiding nausea and vomiting and ways to maintain adequate fluid and food intake. (See box in Tab 3, page 47.)
- Discourage use of unprescribed medications.
- If dehydration or ketosis is present, consider parenteral administration of fluids, electrolytes, and calories. Arrange for appropriate follow-up.

Inadequate Nutrient Intake

- By the first visit in the second trimester, provide counseling to improve the woman's diet. Recommend vitamin/mineral supplementation in addition to improved diet for women with inadequate intakes or unusually high requirements. (For guidance, see the "Indications for Nutrient Supplementation" chart in Tab 1.)

Inappropriate Weight Gain

- If weight gain is below or above the target range, explore possible reasons. (See the box on slow or on rapid weight gain, pages 64 and 65, respectively.)
- Suggest strategies to adjust food intake, if appropriate.

4 Follow-up Visits

Anemia

- Treat iron-deficiency anemia with approximately 60 to 120 mg of ferrous iron daily. At a different time of day, give supplemental zinc and copper as part of a vitamin/mineral supplement. (See Tab 9 for details.)

Side Effects from Iron Supplements

- Side effects are dose related and are most common at doses of 120 mg of elemental iron or more.
- Nausea, cramps, constipation, or diarrhea, if they occur, often persist no longer than 3 to 5 days after the woman begins to take iron supplements. If they do persist, lower the dose temporarily or substitute a slow-release preparation at mealtime.

Suggest, as appropriate:

- *Let me give you the name of a liquid or chewable preparation if you have difficulty swallowing tablets.*
- *Taking iron to treat iron-deficiency anemia helps to reduce fatigue, headache, dizziness, and shortness of breath and increases your ability to adapt to blood loss at the time of delivery.*
- *You may notice a darkening in the color of your stools. High doses of iron sometimes cause constipation or (less often) diarrhea.*
- *Use safety caps and keep supplements out of the reach of children.*

For the Pregnant Woman:

Heartburn

- Eat small, low-fat meals, and eat slowly.
- Take low-fat snacks such as melba toast or fruit as needed for extra energy and nutrients.
- Drink fluids mainly between meals.
- Go easy on spices.
- Avoid lying down for 1 to 2 hours after eating or drinking, especially before going to bed.
- Wear loose-fitting clothing.

Constipation

- Drink 2 to 3 quarts of fluids daily. This includes water, milk, juice, and soup. Warm or hot fluids are especially helpful right after you get up.
- Eat high-fiber cereals and generous amounts of other whole grains, legumes, fruits, and vegetables.
- Take part in physical activities such as walking and swimming.
- Avoid taking laxatives unless recommended by your health care provider.

Positive Glucose Screen

- Perform diagnostic testing for diabetes mellitus.
- If the woman is diagnosed as having gestational diabetes mellitus, complement medical care by the physician by consulting with or arranging for a referral to a dietitian for diet counseling. Such a referral is especially important if insulin therapy is begun.

For the Health Professional:

What to Look for If Weight Gain Is Slow or If Weight Loss Occurs

- Is there a measurement or recording error?
- Is the overall pattern acceptable? Was a lack of gain preceded by a higher than expected gain?
- Was there evidence of edema at the last visit and is it resolved?
- Is nausea, vomiting, or diarrhea a problem?
- Is there a problem with access to food?
- Have psychosocial problems led to poor appetite?
- Does the woman resist weight gain? Is she restricting her energy intake? Does she have an eating disorder?
- If the slow weight gain appears to be a result of self-imposed restriction, does she understand the relationship between her weight gain and her infant's growth and health?
- Is she smoking? How much?
- Is she using alcohol or drugs (especially cocaine or amphetamines)?
- Does her energy expenditure exceed her energy intake?
- Does she have an infection or illness that requires treatment?

For the Health Professional:

What to Look for If Weight Gain Is Very Rapid

- Is there a measurement or recording error?
- Is the overall pattern acceptable? Was the gain preceded by weight loss or a lower than expected gain?
- Is there evidence of edema?
- Has the woman stopped smoking recently? The advantages of smoking cessation offset any disadvantages associated by gaining some extra weight.
- Are twins or triplets a possibility? (A large increase in fundal height may be the earliest sign.)
- Are there signs of gestational diabetes?
- Has there been a dramatic decrease in physical activity without an accompanying decrease in food intake?
- Has the woman greatly increased her food intake? (Get a diet recall, making special note of high-fat foods. However, rapid weight gain is often accompanied by normal eating patterns, which should be continued. If intake of high-fat or high-sugar foods is excessive, encourage substitutions.)
- If serious overeating is occurring, explore why. (Stress? Depression? Eating disorder? Boredom?) Is there a need for special support or a referral?

Pica

- Determine the extent of the practice and its potential for harmful effects.
- If indicated, explore ways to curb or completely eliminate the practice. Guidelines appear in the box.

Bed Rest

- If bed rest is advised, emphasize the importance of achieving adequate energy and nutrient intake for the growth of the fetus, even though the mother's activity level is low. Provide anticipatory guidance. (See box on the next page.) Expect weight fluctuations.
- Arrange for a referral for home health care or homemaker services if indicated.

For the Health Professional:

Pica

Identify pica practices that may be harmful because they interfere with the ingestion of adequate amounts of food, they may lead to intestinal obstruction or impaction, or they may involve toxic substances. Explore possible substitutions for pica substances and behaviors with the woman.

- **When you feel the urge to eat X, what else could you do instead? Take a short walk? Read to your child?**
- **Would you try chewing sugarless gum when you get the urge to eat X?**
- **Instead of chewing ice, try freezing fruit juice cubes to chew.**

For the Pregnant Woman:

Eating Well When on Bed Rest

When on bed rest, planning helps you get the energy and nutrients needed to help your baby grow. If problems arise, the dietitian can give you some practical advice.

Shopping

- Prepare a grocery list for the person who will shop for you or that you can call in to a store that delivers.
- Choose nutritious foods that are easy to eat, easy to prepare or ready to eat, enjoyable cold or at room temperature, and not messy. Convenient choices include individual cans, bottles, or boxes of juice; pieces of fresh fruit; heat-and-serve (microwave) dinners; sandwiches; hard-boiled eggs; nuts; and cheese, milk, and other dairy products.
- To help avoid constipation, include some high-fiber foods like whole grains and fruits and vegetables.
- Try nutritious take-out foods such as pizza, salads, grilled chicken, and burritos.
- Avoid eating fried foods. You are likely to feel more comfortable and to meet your nutrient needs better.

Keeping Food at Your Bedside

- Keep a pitcher of water handy. You need lots of fluids.
- Keep an ice chest nearby for cold drinks and snacks such as milk, cottage cheese, yogurt, fruit juices, sandwiches, cheese, cut-up raw vegetables, and sliced fruit. Keep perishable foods cold.
- Keep whole-grain crackers or bread and peanut butter within reach.

Stimulating Your Appetite

- Make eating enjoyable: plan for variety and for attractive color and texture combinations; eat meals with family or friends.
- Eat small amounts often.

4 Follow-up Visits

5
Postpartum Visits

Checklist

This checklist covers the mother's nutrition and breastfeeding.

In the Hospital

Gathering Information

- [ ] Review the medical record: Medications? Evidence of substance use? Twins? Infant with complications?
- [ ] Need for birth control?
- [ ] Support at home?
- [ ] If breastfeeding, need for special assistance?

Basic Guidance

All Women

- [ ] Dietary Guidelines
- [ ] Appropriate weight change
- [ ] Discharge advice: follow-up, avoidance of harmful substances, adequate rest

Breastfeeding Women

- [ ] Assistance with initiating breastfeeding
- [ ] Additional nutrient, fluid, and energy needs
- [ ] Cautions concerning potentially harmful substances
- [ ] Guidance for successful breastfeeding

Addressing Problems

☐ Facilitate improved access to food
☐ Treat anemia: For iron deficiency—60 to 120 mg of elemental iron daily; also 15 mg of zinc and 2 mg of copper given as part of a vitamin/mineral supplement
☐ Provide support for breastfeeding under challenging circumstances (neonatal complications, multiple gestation, etc.)

Early Pediatric Visit—Maternal Issues

Gathering Information

☐ General: Rest? Eating? Taking liquids?
☐ Breastfeeding experience?
☐ Future plans?

Basic Guidance

☐ Support for breastfeeding
☐ Healthful diet with ample fluids to prevent thirst

Visit at 4 to 6 Weeks Post Partum

Gathering Information

☐ Diet and weight
☐ Breastfeeding

Basic Guidance

☐ Dietary Guidelines with increased intake of milk products, fluids, and foods rich in vitamin A if breastfeeding
☐ Support for breastfeeding
☐ Encouragement of physical activity

Addressing Problems

☐ Counsel how to correct inappropriate weight gain or loss
☐ Discourage restrictive food practices during lactation
☐ Follow up on gestational diabetes mellitus
☐ Combat the use of harmful substances

Postpartum Visits

This section is organized by the timing of the contact with the health care provider and by the woman's lactation status (whether she is breastfeeding or not). It focuses on the woman, not the baby. Ideally, contacts with the mother occur during hospitalization after delivery, within a few days after discharge (a telephone or home visit), at early pediatric visits, and at the visit 4 to 6 weeks post partum. It is highly desirable for all women, regardless of their breastfeeding status, to strive for a healthful diet to replenish nutrient stores and maintain health.

Breastfeeding is the recommended feeding method for infants under ordinary circumstances. Therefore, the establishment of lactation and maintenance of successful breastfeeding are nutritionally relevant to both the mother and her infant. This section includes basic information about breastfeeding. For more detailed sources of information, see Tab 10.

Beginning at delivery and during the first 2 weeks afterward, the nutritional focus of the visits is to establish successful breastfeeding and provide dietary guidance. Support services for breastfeeding mothers should be provided in the hospital. (Short, well-targeted videotapes can be effective and efficient as a part of such an effort.) An early office visit, a visit to the home by a trained health professional, or telephone counseling is often advisable for breastfeeding women.

Later, more attention is directed toward the mother's concerns about the adequacy of her milk supply, healthful weight loss strategies, her return to work or school, and birth control. During follow-up health maintenance visits for the infant and at the postpartum visit for the mother, the health care provider can help to maintain or improve the breastfeeding experience.

Postpartum Nutritional Care in the Hospital

Gathering Information

Check the medical record to identify relevant questions and avoid unnecessary repetition.

- Was the delivery by cesarean section?
- Was it a multiple birth?

History—Sample Questions

General

- *How will your family, friends, or others help you when you go home?*
- *Do you need birth control?*

Breastfeeding

- Does the mother wish to breastfeed? If yes, determine the following by reviewing the mother's history and by physical examination:
  - Is the infant able to latch on to the nipple and areola and suckle vigorously?
  - Are the nipples [still] inverted or flat?
  - Has she been using any medication or drug that is contraindicated when breastfeeding?
  - Does the baby have anomalies or medical complications that may interfere with feeding?

Explanations

All mothers have increased nutritional needs related to pregnancy and childbirth. Women are more likely to be successful at breastfeeding if they receive assistance with breastfeeding basics, relieving engorgement, appropriate birth control methods, and special situations. Combined estrogen and progestin pills may reduce milk volume and the duration of breastfeeding; progestin-only pills have not been found to have this effect.[2]

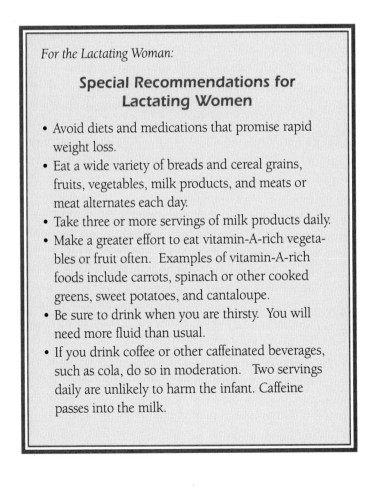

For the Lactating Woman:

Special Recommendations for Lactating Women

- Avoid diets and medications that promise rapid weight loss.
- Eat a wide variety of breads and cereal grains, fruits, vegetables, milk products, and meats or meat alternates each day.
- Take three or more servings of milk products daily.
- Make a greater effort to eat vitamin-A-rich vegetables or fruit often. Examples of vitamin-A-rich foods include carrots, spinach or other cooked greens, sweet potatoes, and cantaloupe.
- Be sure to drink when you are thirsty. You will need more fluid than usual.
- If you drink coffee or other caffeinated beverages, such as cola, do so in moderation. Two servings daily are unlikely to harm the infant. Caffeine passes into the milk.

Basic Guidance

All Women

Diet

- Encourage a healthful diet based on the Dietary Guidelines and suggest eating meals and snacks that are easy to prepare.
- Provide information on the usual pattern of post-partum weight loss.

Discharge Advice

- Arrange for telephone follow-up or a home visit within a few days after hospital discharge to offer support and answer questions.
- *Try to avoid or drastically reduce the use of potentially harmful substances.*
- *Try to rest as much as possible during the day when the baby is sleeping.*
- Schedule the first pediatric visit for the mother and baby 7 to 14 days after delivery, or earlier if discharge from the hospital occurs within 48 hours of delivery.
- Provide guidance for resuming physical activity that considers the mother's current health status.

Breastfeeding Women

Initiating Breastfeeding

- Assist with the initiation of breastfeeding immediately or as soon as possible after delivery. Advise the mother as to positioning, breastfeeding techniques, and removing the infant from the breast.
- *Breastfeed your infant when there are signs of hunger. Feed until at least one breast softens. It is okay to feed on both breasts for as long and as*

often as your baby wants, provided that attachment has been checked to avoid sore nipples. Sometimes feedings will be only about 1 1/2 hours apart.

- Foster a rooming-in situation in the hospital.
- Discourage the hospital staff from giving any supplemental feedings or water.
- Reassure: **Your diet does not have to be "perfect" to nourish your baby well.**
- **The more your baby nurses, the more milk you will produce.**

Diet

- *Take enough fluids (especially milk, juice, water, and soup) to keep from getting thirsty.*
- *You need enough food (at least 1,800 kcal/day) to help maintain milk production and to provide the nutrients that you and your baby need.*
- *For the first 6 weeks, the best guide to how much you should be eating is your own appetite.*
- *Try to keep your intake of coffee, cola, or other sources of caffeine to 2 servings or less per day.*
- Advise against alcohol consumption, and inform the mother that drinking beer does not aid lactation.
- For those who choose to take alcoholic beverages, advise: **It is best to avoid drinking alcoholic beverages, but certainly have no more than 2 to 2.5 oz of liquor, 8 oz of table wine, or 2 cans of beer on any one day** (less for small women).
- If environmental contaminants (e.g., heavy metals such as mercury and organic chemicals such as pesticides) are a potential problem in the area, be on the alert for official advisories concerning foods or areas to avoid.
- If the mother wishes to use beverages containing sugar substitutes, suggest moderation and discourage her from using these to replace important sources of nutrients.

Discharge Advice

- Encourage breastfeeding exclusively for 4 to 6 months.
- *The amount of milk you produce depends directly on how often and how long your baby nurses. A reasonable goal is to nurse the baby whenever he or she is hungry. This may occur 10 or more times per 24 hours during the first few weeks after birth. Newborns who sleep for more than 3 to 4 hours may need to be awakened for feeding if they are not gaining weight and have little urine and stool output.*
- *You know your baby is getting milk if milk leaks from the alternate breast when you're nursing, you hear your baby swallow, or the baby has six to eight wet diapers and at least one dirty diaper a day.*
- *Relax and find a comfortable place to feed, and enjoy your baby.*
- *Avoid supplemental feedings of formula or water.*
- Discuss strategies for maintaining healthy breasts: frequent nursing, proper positioning, using a finger to break suction before removing the infant from the breast, and identification of early signs of mastitis to permit rapid treatment. Explain that some nipple tenderness may occur at the beginning of the feed during the first 2 weeks but that it is usually not long lasting.
- Teach all breastfeeding mothers how to express milk manually. Demonstrate the use of pumps if indicated.
- Reaffirm that the mother is doing something really important for her baby.
- If a multivitamin/mineral supplement was prescribed during pregnancy, consider continued use of it during lactation. (See supplement chart, Tab 1.)
- Check the mother's understanding of instructions about getting help with breastfeeding if questions or problems arise.

Addressing Problems

All Women

Suspected Difficulty in Obtaining Adequate Food

- Refer mother to food assistance programs such as WIC and food stamps. (See Tab 10.)

Postpartum Anemia

- Check for postpartum anemia if there was unusually heavy blood loss at delivery. If detected, start a therapeutic dose of iron of 60 to 120 mg/day. At a different time of day, give 15 mg of zinc and 2 mg of copper as part of a vitamin/mineral supplement. Recheck hemoglobin or hematocrit at the mother's 6-week postpartum visit.

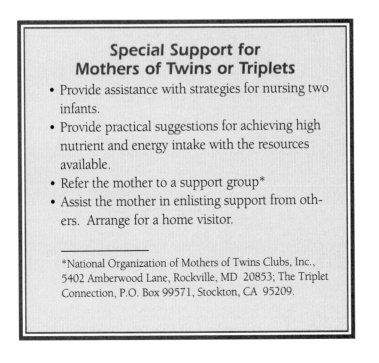

Special Support for Mothers of Twins or Triplets

- Provide assistance with strategies for nursing two infants.
- Provide practical suggestions for achieving high nutrient and energy intake with the resources available.
- Refer the mother to a support group*
- Assist the mother in enlisting support from others. Arrange for a home visitor.

---

*National Organization of Mothers of Twins Clubs, Inc., 5402 Amberwood Lane, Rockville, MD 20853; The Triplet Connection, P.O. Box 99571, Stockton, CA 95209.

Breastfeeding Women

Lack of Support for Breastfeeding

- Provide support and/or refer to a local support resource.

Low Birth Weight Baby or Other Neonatal Complications

- Consult with the team member who is an expert in breastfeeding management for advice and information about special care, such as:
  - Establishing and maintaining lactation.
  - Safe storage of mother's milk.
  - Support and encouragement for the mother.

Cesarean Delivery

- Help the mother find comfortable positions (e.g., lying down, using pillows) for breastfeeding.
- Initiate breastfeeding as soon as the mother and infant are ready.
- Minimize interrupting the mother's sleep for reasons other than breastfeeding.
- Assist the mother in enlisting support from family, friends, or support groups such as La Leche League.

Breast Surgery or Anatomical Variants

- If an anatomical variation was not corrected prenatally, consult an experienced clinician for observation and assessment of breastfeeding and for guidance in using a breast pump or breast shells to evert the nipples.
- Facilitate nursing after delivery.
- Encourage women with previous breast augmentation or reduction to monitor the infant's weight gain regularly.

Smoking and Use of Contraindicated Drugs

- Encourage mothers who smoke to stop smoking and help them to do so. **Be sure not to smoke while nursing the baby.**
- If the mother has been using illicit mood-altering drugs, recommendations concerning breastfeeding should be made, on a case-by-case basis, by the health care team.
- Drugs that are contraindicated during breastfeeding include bromocriptine, cocaine, cyclophosphamide, cyclosporine, doxorubicin, ergotamine, lithium, methotrexate, phencyclidine (PCP), and phenindione (not used in the United States).[16]
- Radiopharmaceuticals that require temporary cessation of breastfeeding include gallium-67, indium-111, iodine-125, iodine-131, radioactive sodium, and technetium-99m.[16]
- If the mother wishes to breastfeed after treatment with a contraindicated drug is discontinued, assist her with pumping her breasts to maintain lactation and explain why the milk must be discarded.
- Request consultation concerning safe medically indicated drugs for use when breastfeeding. (See Study Group on Human Lactation and Breastfeeding, under "Examples of Breastfeeding Projects to Assist Health Professionals," Tab 10.)

Early Pediatric Visit

The first baby visit provides an opportunity to ask the mother about her diet and home situation and about how breastfeeding is going.

Gathering Information

Physical Examination

- Measure the infant's weight and length, and record measurements on the growth chart as a means of evaluating the infant's nutrition.
- Observe the mother nursing the baby, if applicable, noting the method of holding the infant, the infant's ability to latch on and suckle, the removal of the infant from the breast, signs that the mother is comfortable, and her responses.

History—Sample Questions

General

- *How are things going at home?*
- *Are you enjoying your baby?*
- *How much sleep (rest) are you getting?*
- *Do you have trouble finding time to eat? To drink enough liquids? How often are you eating and drinking? Any snacks? What liquids are you drinking?* If she is eating fewer than three meals per day, get more details.
- *How are you feeding your baby?*

Breastfeeding Experience

If the woman is breastfeeding, ask:

- *How often are you breastfeeding your baby?*
- *How are you doing with breastfeeding?*

- *Are your breasts comfortable now? Your nipples? What, if anything, are you feeding your baby besides your milk? Why? How often? When?*
- *About how much has your weight changed since you left the hospital?*

Future Plans

- *How long do you plan to breastfeed?*
- *Do you plan to go to work or school? If so, when?*
- *Tell me how you will combine work and breast-feeding. Perhaps I can make some suggestions about feeding your baby while you're at work, expressing milk, storing milk, and managing on days off from work.*

Explanations

Physical Examination

Slow infant growth may be a sign that the mother needs assistance with breastfeeding or with formula feeding. Early identification and correction of positioning problems may promote continuation of breastfeeding.

General

Support and care for the primary caretaker and family will assist in optimal care of the infant. The mother benefits from help to meet her own needs for rest and a healthful diet.

Breastfeeding Experience

Most problems with breastfeeding the neonate can be resolved through relatively simple measures such as feeding on demand, proper positioning, breastfeeding exclusively (without feeding formula or other supplements), pumping the breasts if absences are unavoidable, alternating the breasts, and releasing suction when removing the infant from the breast.

Basic Guidance

- Reassure the mother, as appropriate, and reinforce her successes, such as the infant's growth or the feeding relationship.
- *You can expect your baby to want to nurse more often if he or she starts to have a growth spurt. This will increase your milk supply.*
- Discuss strategies and provide materials to assist in coping with the demands of the newborn and other family members.
- If applicable, provide tips for eating well with fewer calories (see ideas on page 108 and "Boosting Your Nutrient Intake," page 103.
- Encourage the mother to consume a healthful diet based mainly on the Dietary Guidelines (see "Basic Dietary Guidance," Tab 2).
- Discourage her from trying diets and drugs that promise quick weight loss.
- Provide information for the mother or primary meal preparer concerning practical strategies for healthful family meals.
- Assist the mother in finding valid answers to her breastfeeding questions.

Addressing Problems

- Check on the mother's need for physician referral to a breastfeeding specialist.
- For problem resolution for breastfeeding mothers, see Tab 10 for sources of information.

Visit at 4 to 6 Weeks Post Partum

The customary postpartum visit with the obstetric care provider offers a valuable opportunity to assess problems relating to the mother's nutritional status and breastfeeding experience.

Gathering Information

History—Sample Questions

General

- *How many hours of sleep are you able to get?*
- *Have you gone to work outside your home or to school?* If not, *Are you planning to do so?*

Diet and Weight

- *How many times a day do you eat?*
- *About how many glasses or cups of fluids are you drinking every day?*
- *How do you feel about your weight now?*
- If the mother is concerned about excessive weight, ask: *Are you trying to lose weight? How? What is your weight loss goal?*

Breastfeeding

- *Are you continuing to breastfeed your baby?*
  If mother is breastfeeding with or without supplementary formula, ask:
  - *How many times a day do you breastfeed your baby?*
  - *When do you alternate your breasts?*
  - *How is breastfeeding going for you?*

- *Are you avoiding any foods because you are nursing? Which ones?*
- *May I offer some suggestions for combining work with breastfeeding?*
- *Are you using some kind of birth control?*
  If yes, ask: **What method?**
  If no, ask: **Do you need birth control?**

Physical Examination

- Examine breasts.
- Measure weight.

Explanations

History

General

Some mothers need assistance to find practical strategies for getting adequate rest and resuming outside activities, expecially if they are breastfeeding.

Diet and Weight

Some mothers benefit from concrete suggestions for achieving adequate intake in the face of increased family demands. The use of rapid weight-loss methods should be discouraged. Weight loss is usually gradual; it may take many months to achieve prepregnant weight. Some women resume smoking to lose weight more easily, but this poses long-term health risks for the mother, exposes the infant to smoke, and may interfere with the let-down reflex when nursing.

Breastfeeding

Infrequent or delayed feeding may lead to problems of reduced milk supply and engorgement. Problems with nipples may lead to reduced frequency of feeding. Avoidance of specific foods by the mother seldom benefits the baby. Combined estrogen and progestin pills may reduce milk volume and the duration of breastfeeding; progestin-only pills have not been found to have this effect.[2]

Physical Examination

Rapid weight loss often occurs over the first month post partum without restricting food intake, regardless of breastfeeding status. Engorged breasts and cracked nipples signal a need for support with breastfeeding.

Basic Guidance

All Women

- Encourage a healthful diet based on the Dietary Guidelines (see "Basic Dietary Guidance," Tab 2, page 27).
- Assist the mother or primary meal preparer with strategies for a healthful diet for the family.
- Clarify that (further) weight loss will occur only if energy intake is less than energy expenditure (plus the energy content of the milk produced).
- Discourage the use of harmful substances.
- Encourage physical activity.

Breastfeeding Women

- Encourage generous intake of milk products, fluids, and foods rich in vitamin A. (See box "Special Recommendations for Lactating Women," page 73.)
- Explain that most women who breastfeed can eat more calories than they could before pregnancy without gaining weight.
- Answer questions concerning breastfeeding.

For the Health Professional:

Signals of Possible Weight-Related Problems During Lactation

Consider diet counseling for women if any of the following applies:

All Breastfeeding Women

- Abnormally slow infant growth despite frequent feedings and other appropriate breastfeeding techniques.

Women with Normal Prepregnancy Weight for Height

- Weight loss in excess of 4.5 lb (approximately 2 kg)/month after the first month post partum.
- Weight falling below normal weight for height.
- Weight gain leading to high weight for height.
- Preoccupation with weight combined with major fluctuations in weight. (Look for additional signs of an eating disorder.)

Women with Low Prepregnancy Weight for Height

- Any weight loss after weight for height returns to the low prepregnancy weight-for-height category (or after the weight returns to the prepregnancy weight).
- Weight loss in excess of 4.5 lb (approximately 2 kg)/month after the first month post partum.

Women with High or Very High Prepregnancy Weight for Height

- Weight loss in excess of 6.5 lb (approximately 3 kg)/month after the first month post partum.
- Postpartum weight gain.

Addressing Problems

Weight Problems

- Determine possible causes of excessive postpartum weight loss, weight gain, or lack of any weight loss (see box); and check on the infant's growth.
- Counsel the woman about strategies to adjust her energy and nutrient intakes, alter her level of physical activity, or both.
- Recommend a low-dose multivitamin/mineral supplement (this can be the same as the prenatal supplement) if the mother has been curbing energy intake excessively and is unlikely to increase her nutrient intake.

Restrictive Food Practices During Lactation

If a breastfeeding mother is restricting her food intake to prevent colic, allergic reactions, or other problems in her infant, tell her that the evidence does not support *routine* elimination of milk or other basic foods to prevent these problems. If symptoms are serious, it may be advisable to demonstrate objectively whether food avoidance will help, as outlined below.

- Remove the suspected food allergen from the mother's diet. (This may require diet counseling.)
- Determine if the infant becomes asymptomatic.
- If yes, conduct an oral challenge under careful medical supervision to determine whether the symptoms recur.
- Treat provoked reactions appropriately.

If the mother must eliminate a basic food from her diet for weeks to months, provide for diet counseling to promote adequate nutrient intake.

Glucose Intolerance

- For those who developed gestational diabetes, follow up on current glucose tolerance.
- Consider providing or refer for weight control counseling as appropriate to reduce the risk of developing type II diabetes mellitus.

Use of Harmful Substances

- Assist women who smoke cigarettes, use smokeless tobacco, abuse alcohol, or use illegal drugs to quit. Include diet counseling to address their concerns about weight, as appropriate.
- Refer women to evaluation or treatment programs as needed.

II Supplementary Information

6
General Strategies for Providing Effective Nutritional Care

Essential Steps for Patient Education

1. Identify the problem, such as inadequate weight gain, using information from the nutrition assessment.

2. Develop a tentative clinical objective to discuss with the woman. The objective should be based on clinical standards and information obtained from screening and assessment procedures. An example would be to gain at least 3 lb by the next visit (in 1 month).

3. Determine the woman's perception of the seriousness of the problem (e.g., inadequate weight gain) and the likelihood it will harm her or her baby.

4. If the woman does not believe that the problem is serious or that it applies to her, offer personalized information to help her to see this as a problem for her, e.g., small babies may look cuter and be easier to deliver, but they are much more likely to get sick.

5. Decide which behavior(s) supports or impedes the achievement of the clinical objective. Try to identify more than one behavior (e.g., decrease exercise, increase intake of foods high in energy and nutrients, and take specific actions to decrease stress) to give the woman choices.

6. With the woman, assess the barriers to behavior change and find strategies to overcome them, based on the woman's own experience and the experience of people who influence her. Consider asking her to list the benefits to her and her baby.

7. Negotiate with the woman about which behavior change(s) is to be attempted. It is best to begin with small changes in one or two behaviors that the woman will be able to make and maintain. Personalize the benefits of behavior change by relating them to concerns she has expressed and by using language forms such as "you," "your baby."

8. Help to reduce barriers. For example, refer the woman for special counseling or to food assistance agencies, provide appropriate written material, or loan the family a videotape. Improve support by family and friends by offering assistance from the staff or volunteers.

9. Offer feedback and reinforce *any* success. When there is little or no progress, step up the frequency of contact (e.g., by telephone) and use more specialized resources.

Responding to Developmental Differences

Adolescents pose special challenges to health care providers because of the need to be aware of and responsive to their developmental differences. Depending on her developmental stage, one adolescent of a given age may need to be approached very differently from another. The following chart provides a brief summary of some useful approaches by stage rather than age.

	Stages of Adolescence		
	Early	Middle	Late
Goal-setting ability of the teen	Limited—may be unable to formulate goals, or the goals may be unrealistic.	Improving, but still limited—may formulate grandiose, unrealistic goals.	Often able to make realistic plans for the future, but may not be interested or willing to do so.
Useful professional approaches	Be caring yet firm. Offer simple, concrete choices. Encourage causal reasoning. Offer positive reinforcement, and build the teen's self-esteem.	Be caring and demonstrate respect for the teen's need to make decisions independently as well as to conform to peer pressures, but set limits firmly. Encourage negotiation with adults and assist in learning negotiation skills. Encourage consideration of the possible consequences of acts and the formation of realistic goals.	Be caring and be a good listener. Offer opinions as one adult to another. Serve as a resource and a sounding board.

Adapted from Department of Pediatrics, University of Rochester, as seen in *A Smart Start: Nutrition for Life.*[17]

Serving Culturally Diverse Populations*

A basic element of culturally appropriate care is demonstrating a sincere commitment to providing services in an acceptable and appropriate manner to people of cultural or ethnic groups different from one's own. Since cultural groups may differ in many ways, considering some of the questions and approaches listed below may help to achieve this. Attentive listening helps the care provider learn.

- *Definition of family and of the roles of family members.* Is it a nuclear family unit? Is it an extended family? If extended, how many members and generations are included (grandparents, aunts and uncles)? How are decisions made within the family? (Does the male play a dominant role? The grandmother?)
- *Childrearing practices.* Is child care shared as a method of extending the family's resources? Does the grandmother care for the infant soon after birth so that the mother can earn an income or return to school?
- *Beliefs and practices concerning health and illness.* Does religion play a role? Is balance between dichotomies such as "hot" and "cold" or "yin" and "yang" believed to contribute to health? If so, how can balance be achieved, and how is this likely to affect food selection? Are certain foods viewed as healthful or harmful during pregnancy or lactation? Is there a belief that eating too much or taking supplements will lead to difficult labor and delivery?
- *Styles of interaction between professionals and group members.* Do group members tend to prefer a warm, friendly, and personal form of communication or a more formal one? How important is the use of formal titles? Do group members tend to prefer to sit or stand closer to or farther away from

---

*Much of the content of this section was derived from Anderson and Fenichel.[18]

Elements of Culturally Effective Programs

Basic elements of a program to promote culturally appropriate care include the following:

- In-service training of the health care providers on the cultural practices and beliefs of the groups served.
- Creation of a welcoming environment and use of materials that portray a positive image of the clientele.
- Employment of health care providers who are members of the cultural groups served or well-trained interpreters.
- Development of a mechanism for input from the community, making certain that all cultural groups are represented.

the provider than the provider is used to? Does direct eye contact facilitate communication or does it signal disrespect? Is touching the person viewed as offensive or as an important means of communication? Is it important to address elders first?

- *Orientation toward the future or the present.* Is there a tendency to live in the present with little regard for the future? Is education viewed as such an important key to the future that it takes priority over other activities?
- *Dietary practices. What foods form the basis for the group's diet?* What are the key sources of essential nutrients? Do any customary cooking methods enhance the quality of diet? Useful sources of information about local dietary practices are usually available from the state department of health or the state WIC office.

- *Ways in which foods are integrated into the diet.* Are vegetables added to soups, stews, rice, or other dishes instead of eaten as a side dish or in salads? Is milk used as the liquid in cooked cereal, blended with fruit, or mixed half and half with coffee or tea rather than being used alone as a beverage?

Extending the Effectiveness of Nutrition Education Through Trained Peer Counselors

Trained peer counselors afford a means to extend the reach and effectiveness of health care providers—especially for breastfeeding women, members of ethnic minorities, and adolescents. Women who have successfully implemented nutritional recommendations as patients are candidates for the special training required.

Prior to the encounter between the woman and the provider, the peer counselor may meet with the woman to review objectives from the previous visit and the extent to which they were met, determine the woman's nutrition- or health-related concerns, review topics that are scheduled to be discussed during the visit, and help the woman develop appropriate questions based on her needs.

Following the encounter between the woman and the provider, the peer counselor may meet with the woman to review what was discussed, determine whether the instructions are understood, help her make plans based on available resources, alert her to resources to improve her nutritional status, and encourage her to follow up and to take responsibility for her own health and welfare.

As needed, the peer counselor may provide other services, including giving food demonstrations and helping design educational materials.

7
Dietary Assessment and Guidance

Dietary assessment is one of several key elements of overall nutrition assessment. (The other elements include assessment of weight status, laboratory values, and clinical data.) Some approaches to the collection of dietary data are very easy for any practitioner; others require a high degree of skill.

Standard Approaches for Assessing Intake

In a *diet* or *food recall,* the woman is asked to recall everything she ate and drank within a specified period, usually 24 hours. Diet recalls are usually easy to obtain if only qualitative information is sought about foods eaten on the previous day. A few simple questions will usually help spark a flagging memory. Often there is no need to probe for accompaniments or portion size. These details are most important in relation to problems with weight or disease conditions. Because food intake fluctuates from day to day, it is important to try to ascertain whether the intakes on the day reported were typical or whether they reflected unusual intake because of illness, a party, or another infrequent event.

In a *food frequency questionnaire,* the woman is asked how often she ate the foods on the list over a specified period, usually one week or longer. Food frequency questionnaires help identify the core diet and how it can be built upon. For example, a woman who eats soup daily could be encouraged to add vegetables to it. The questionnaires also provide a summary of the foods used over a period of time. They can be used to identify women who seldom eat important nutrient sources, who never eat any foods from a food group, or who eat large amounts of foods high in calories and low in essential nutrients. Some can be scored readily by computer. Although some women appear to have difficulty understanding the concepts involved in a food frequency questionnaire and may grossly overreport their food intake, the questionnaire may be helpful in identifying foods that the woman is willing to eat and thus useful in diet counseling.

For *food* or *diet records,* women are asked to record names and amounts of all the foods and beverages they consumed for a specified period (e.g., 1 day, 3 days, or 1 week). Food or diet records are potentially accurate sources of dietary information, especially if the woman has considerable writing and recording skill and has been trained in how to measure portion sizes and keep the records. Since recording food intake may lead to changes in eating behavior, the practice should be monitored to reinforce desirable behaviors and to avoid adverse effects (such as inadequate weight gain during pregnancy). Records may be most useful for obtaining quantitative information relative to modified diets or for identifying behaviors that might be improved.

In a *checklist,* such as the one in the nutrition questionnaire, pages 7 and 8, the woman is asked to mark which of the listed foods she ate during a specified period. Checklists are easy for most people to complete, and they provide an informative glimpse of dietary practices. For illiterate women, realistic pictures or drawings can be used. It is desirable to supplement such forms by asking a few key questions and observing nonverbal communication, as well as by paying careful attention to the oral responses.

Selecting an Approach for Dietary Assessment

To select the appropriate method for a given woman and situation, the following questions may be useful:

- *What is my objective in collecting the information?* Possible objectives include finding out whether the woman has an energy deficit or whether her intake of folate is adequate.
- *How will I use the information?* In other words, how accurate and detailed does the food intake information need to be? Possible uses include determination of the woman's eligibility for participation in WIC, of the need either for counseling to improve diet quality or to take nutrient supplements, and of appropriate food choices or menu patterns. The latter can be used when developing a detailed plan for a modified diet to help with the management of a disease or an inborn error of metabolism. Avoid collecting information that you will not use.
- *What is the standard to which the information collected should be compared—a predetermined number of servings of foods from various food groups or a nutrient standard such as the Recommended Dietary Allowances?*[19] Most often it is sufficient to direct attention to food use rather than to intake of specific nutrients. For example, three servings of milk or cheese daily ensures adequate calcium intake with few exceptions (such as the breastfeeding of twins). Attention to intake of specific nutrients is essential in the management of diabetes mellitus, renal disease, certain gastrointestinal diseases, and phenylketonuria.
- *What resources do I have for collecting, analyzing, and interpreting dietary data?* If there is a need for a detailed dietary assessment to serve as the basis for a modified diet or for intensive diet counseling, the services of a dietitian are highly desirable. For health care practices that do not include a dietitian, arrangements for consultation and referral are needed.

A dietitian can assist in developing routine procedures for dietary assessment and can train other providers to use those procedures proficiently. A dietitian might be located by contacting a local hospital, public health agency, or the state dietetic association.

Some dietary analysis computer software is targeted for use by health care providers, whereas some is targeted for use by clients. If a self-administered program is easy to use and a computer is available, this can be an efficient mechanism for collecting and summarizing dietary data. However, since the outputs from dietary analysis programs can be seriously misinterpreted, it is advisable to consult with a dietitian before obtaining dietary analysis software and implementing its use.

Tips for Dietary Guidance

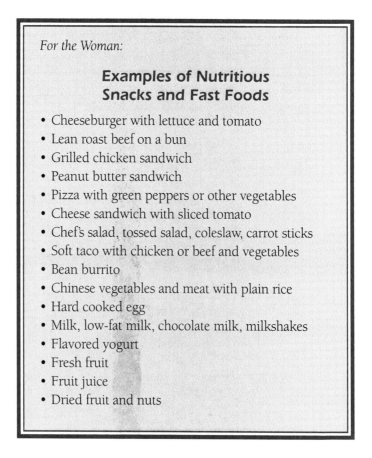

For the Woman:

Examples of Nutritious Snacks and Fast Foods

- Cheeseburger with lettuce and tomato
- Lean roast beef on a bun
- Grilled chicken sandwich
- Peanut butter sandwich
- Pizza with green peppers or other vegetables
- Cheese sandwich with sliced tomato
- Chef's salad, tossed salad, coleslaw, carrot sticks
- Soft taco with chicken or beef and vegetables
- Bean burrito
- Chinese vegetables and meat with plain rice
- Hard cooked egg
- Milk, low-fat milk, chocolate milk, milkshakes
- Flavored yogurt
- Fresh fruit
- Fruit juice
- Dried fruit and nuts

Increasing the Calcium Intake of Women with Lactose Intolerance

Encourage attempts to consume milk products, at least on a trial basis, since lactose tolerance often improves during pregnancy. If milk is not tolerated, be sure to check on the woman's vitamin D status by asking about exposure to sunlight.

- *Try small servings (for example, a small [4 oz] juice glass) of milk several times daily.* Whole milk may be tolerated better than low-fat or skim milk, and taking milk with other foods often helps avoid symptoms.
- *Try yogurt containing active, live cultures. To save money, buy a large container of plain yogurt and stir in fruit and sugar or jam or other flavorings to taste.*
- *Try aged hard cheese such as cheddar cheese.*
- *Try taking lactase tablets or drops when drinking milk. Follow the directions on the package.*
- *Try lactase-treated milk and milk products.* These are more expensive than untreated products. Women who participate in WIC may be able to obtain them through WIC.
- *Try cultured buttermilk for drinking or baking.*

If these strategies are unsuccessful, explore ways to increase calcium intake from foods that contain no milk products such as those listed on the next page. Consider recommending a calcium supplement.

For the Woman:

Ways to Increase Your Calcium Intake If You Avoid Most Milk Products

• Choose more foods that provide calcium, such as the following.

Foods equal to about 1 cup of milk in calcium content:

   3 oz. of sardines (if the bones are eaten)

Foods equal to about ½ cup of milk in calcium content:

   3 oz. of canned salmon (if the bones are eaten)
   4 oz. of tofu (if it has been processed with calcium sulfate)
   4 oz. of collards
   1 waffle* (7 inches in diameter)
   4 corn tortillas (if processed with calcium salts)

Foods equal to about ⅓ cup of milk in calcium content:

   1 cup of cooked dried beans
   4 oz. of bok choy or turnip greens or kale
   1 medium square of cornbread* (2½ × 2½ × 1½ inches)
   2 pancakes* (4 inches in diameter)
   7 to 9 oysters
   3 oz. of shrimp

Foods that can be made high in calcium:

   Soups made from bones cooked with vinegar or tomato
   Macaroni and cheese* and other combination foods made
      with good sources of calcium

• Ask your health care provider about taking a calcium supplement.

*A dairy product is a major contributor to the calcium content of this food.

For the Woman:
Boosting Your Nutrient Intake

Substitute similar foods that provide more nutrients for the calories, for example:

Foods That Are Low in Vitamins and Minerals	Foods That Are Higher in Vitamins and Minerals
Bologna	Sliced chicken
Bacon	Ham
Cake	Ice milk, pudding
Fruit drinks	Fruit juices
Jello®	Fresh fruit

Choose lower-calorie versions of the same foods to make room for good nutrient sources, for example:

Commonly Eaten Food	Lower-Calorie Version
Ice cream	Ice milk or frozen yogurt
Whole milk	Low-fat or skim milk
Fried chicken	Grilled chicken or fried chicken without the skin
American cheese	Low-fat cheese
Cream soup	Vegetable soup
Choice or prime beef	Lean beef
Chips	Unbuttered popcorn, pretzels

Cut back on foods high in calories, such as those listed below, to make room for foods that are better sources of vitamins and minerals.

High-Calorie Foods That Are Low in Essential Nutrients

Most deep-fried foods and fat-rich foods (such as onion rings, fried taco shells, chips, doughnuts, bacon, and sausages)
Soft drinks, Kool-Aid®, and fruit punch.
Salad dressings and mayonnaise
Most desserts (such as cookies, cakes, and pies)
Fats and oils
Most sweets (such as candy, sugar, and honey)

For the Health Professional:

Special Concerns for Some Low-Income Women

Problem	Possible Short-Term Solutions
Local water tastes bad	Encourage the women to bring water jugs to the clinic to fill. Discuss bottled water.
No refrigeration	Explore the possibility of using a cooler with ice or of making a cold box. Suggest nutritious foods that don't require refrigeration, such as peanut butter, bread, fruit, vegetables, and canned foods.
No cooking facilities, homeless	If the woman is on WIC, ask about the special food package for women without cooking facilities; explore potential for use of hot plate; caution against indoor use of charcoal grills.
No money or food stamps to buy food	Recommend food pantries, soup kitchens, or shelters to get meals until food stamps are issued. Assist the woman with obtaining expedited processing of her application for food stamps or for WIC or applying for other assistance programs.
Dependent on home-grown vegetables or wild foods (seasonal)	Explore the possibility of creating an indoor greenhouse; offer information about food preservation and safe food storage or refer to Cooperative Extension.

8
Assessing Weight Change

Procedures for Obtaining Accurate Measurements

Weight

Weigh women on a platform beam balance scale with movable weights or on a high-quality electronic scale that is graduated to the nearest 0.25 lb (100 g), and use the same scale each time.

Be consistent in the amount of clothing allowed during weighing. If weighing must be done in street clothes, it is desirable to ask patients to remove shoes, outer clothing such as sweaters and jackets, and purses.

The person who measures the weight should adopt a nonjudgmental demeanor regarding weight and weight change. If this person comments about a change in weight, that comment and its tone should be consistent with the message being given by all the other health professionals.

Measurement or assessment of the weight of women with disabilities may require alternative approaches. For example, wheelchair-bound women can be weighed using a special wheelchair scale and subtracting the weight of the chair. If such a scale is unavailable, one can be improvised by building two bathroom scales into a frame with a short ramp (each wheel rests on a scale). Or the woman can be weighed by difference if her partner is accustomed to carrying her.

Estimates of weight-for-height status are affected if one or more limbs are missing (a visual impression should be sufficient), but changes in weight are unlikely to be affected if there is no change in any prosthetic device used. (A typical prosthesis weighs approximately 3 to 5 lb [1.5 to 2.5 kg].)

Height

The most accurate method is to measure height before pregnancy or as early in the pregnancy as possible to reduce errors caused by changes in posture. Use a stadiometer, either one constructed at the health center or a commercial one that is not built into a weighing scale. Push the vertical board flat against the wall and lower it along the metal measuring tape until the horizontal board touches the woman's scalp. A less accurate method (but one that is better than self-reported height) is to use a stadiometer that is built into a weighing scale.

Quality Control Measures

To help achieve consistent, accurate measurements by different staff members, four additional steps are recommended:

- Zero the scale daily.
- Calibrate the scale regularly (about once a month). Record the amount of drift.
- Provide in-service training concerning standard procedures for measuring weight and height.
- Monitor measurement techniques regularly.

Promoting Weight Gain

Substantial weight gain is recommended during pregnancy, as shown in the weight gain grid in Tab 1.

Weight gain may also be recommended for very thin women who are not pregnant, especially for those planning a pregnancy.

Identify the Cause of Low Weight Gain

Potential causes include lack of food, concern about body image, poor appetite, prolonged nausea and vomiting, alcohol abuse, excessive activity leading to high energy expenditure or skipping of meals, and health problems.

Questions and suggestions include:

- *Do you need some help in getting enough food to eat?*
  - *Have you picked up your WIC vouchers? Food stamps?*
  - *Were you able to use them?*
- *Take a look at your activity level. Do you need to slow down?*
- *Do you need to set aside or plan more time for meals?*
- *Are you worried about gaining too much weight?*
- *Do some problems at work or home cause you to lose your appetite? Would you like help coping with them?*

Find Solutions

Suggestions include:

- *Eat small amounts frequently. Plan ahead for some nutritious snacks.*
- *Fruit juices, milk, or milkshakes can be good substitutes for noncaloric beverages such as water, coffee, or sugar-free soft drinks.*
- *Whole-grain bread and rolls are quick, tasty, nutritious, and easy to digest.*

- *Here are some places you can go to get some food if you run out . . .* (e.g., a local hunger hotline and food pantry).
- *This is how to enroll in the . . .* (e.g., Expanded Food and Nutrition Education Program [EFNEP]).
- *Let me introduce you to our social worker, who will try to help you obtain some extra assistance.*

Promoting a Lower Rate of Weight Gain

The following suggestions are targeted specifically to pregnant women, but most of them are applicable to nonpregnant women who want to control their weight.

Suggestions include:

- *Be sure to continue to eat foods such as fruits, vegetables, whole-grain breads, low-fat milk, legumes, and lean meat, chicken, or fish.*
- *Aim to gain at the rate shown on your weight gain grid even if you have already gained more than the recommended amount. Your baby still needs to gain weight.*
- *If you gained weight fast because you ate a lot, look for ways to cut back on foods high in fat and sugar. Also try to avoid situations that lead you to overeat.*
- *Club soda or mineral water, plain or mixed with fruit juice, makes a good substitute for soft drinks.*
- *If you are not getting much exercise, what can you do safely to use up more energy? Walk? Swim? Dance?* Even moderate exercise may be contraindicated for women with multiple gestations, cervical incompetence, or certain other complications of pregnancy.

9
Nutrient Supplementation

Identifying Anemia

Blood Sampling

Blood is drawn for analysis of hemoglobin or hematocrit at the preconception/interconception and first prenatal visits. Venipuncture blood yields the most reproducible results and is recommended, in particular, for confirmatory and follow-up studies after anemia has been detected.

The use of skin puncture blood is acceptable but will result in more false-positive and false-negative values. Use of disposable, spring-loaded lancets is helpful. Make the process quick because a few minutes of anxiety results in a cold, sweaty hand and poor blood flow. To improve accuracy, discard the first drop of blood and do not squeeze the finger because this makes tissue fluids contaminate the blood.

Criteria for Anemia

Hemoglobin and hematocrit values are *normally* lower in pregnant than in nonpregnant women, and they reach the lowest values during the second trimester of pregnancy. Anemia should be defined using the appropriate cutoff values from Table 1 or 2 in Tab 1 (page 16), after adjusting the cutoff value for high altitude (see Table 3 on the next page), if applicable. The effects of altitude and smoking are additive.

TABLE 3. Adjustments for Altitudes[a]

Altitude (feet)	Adjustment Value	
	Hemoglobin (g/dl)	Hematocrit (%)
3,000–3,999	+0.2	+0.5
4,000–4,999	+0.3	+1.0
5,000–5,999	+0.5	+1.5
6,000–6,999	+0.7	+2.0

[a]From CDC.[11] To avoid underdiagnosis of anemia at high altitude, add the appropriate value from this table to the cutoff value given in Table 1 or 2 in Tab 1, page 16.

Example: A woman living in Denver at an altitude of 5,280 ft and smoking 15 cigarettes per day would have a cutoff value for anemia of 11.8 g hemoglobin/dl during her first trimester:

11.3 + 0.5 for altitude.

If her hemoglobin were 11.5 g/dl at 11 weeks of gestation, she would be considered anemic.

Indications for Additional Testing

Serum Ferritin. Serum ferritin provides an estimate of iron reserves. Consider analysis of serum ferritin to confirm that an anemia is due to iron deficiency, especially if there has been inadequate or no hemoglobin or hematocrit response to iron supplementation.

Iron Supplements

Iron deficiency is the most common cause of anemia during pregnancy. To prevent iron deficiency anemia, routinely recommend iron supplementation at a low dose, about 30 mg of elemental iron/day, for nonanemic pregnant women during the second and third trimesters. Low-dose iron can be given alone or as part of a multivitamin/mineral supplement of appropriate composition for pregnancy. Effective forms of iron include ferrous sulfate, ferrous fumarate, and ferrous gluconate. Liquid and chewable forms are available for women who have trouble swallowing tablets or capsules. These iron preparations may stain teeth, but the stain can be removed by brushing. Recommend taking the supplement at bedtime or between meals with water or juice, not with milk, tea, or coffee. (Fruit juice will not enhance the absorption of iron from supplements, but some women may be more likely to drink fruit juice if advised to do so with a supplement. On the other hand, it is important for a woman to know that water is fine if juice is not available.)

For anemic women, start a therapeutic dose of about 60 to 120 mg of elemental iron/day. Give 60 mg/day as a single dose or 120 mg/day as two separate doses, between meals and/or at bedtime with water or juice. In addition, to ensure an adequate supply of zinc and copper, recommend a multivitamin/mineral supplement of appropriate composition for pregnancy (see "Suggested Content of Prenatal Vitamin/Mineral Supplements") to be taken with a meal. Side effects of nausea, "stomach" discomfort, constipation, or diarrhea may occur during the first few days. If they persist, try a slow-release iron preparation given with meals. Check the hemoglobin or hematocrit again after 1 month. If the anemia is not improved or resolved, consider other causes of anemia. If the anemia is resolved, lower the dose of iron to 30 mg/day. For sample statements about iron supplements, see page 62.

9 Supplementation

Suggested Content of Prenatal Vitamin/Mineral Supplements

The following is the suggested approximate composition of prenatal multivitamin/mineral supplements for use by women identified to be at high nutritional risk. (See the chart "Indications for Nutrient Supplementation" in Tab 1 for further information.)

Iron	30–60 mg
Zinc	15 mg
Copper	2 mg
Calcium	250 mg
Vitamin D	10 μg (400 IU)
Vitamin C	50 mg
Vitamin B_6	2 mg
Folate	300 μg
Vitamin B_{12}	2 μg

If vitamin A is included, beta-carotene is preferred over retinol to reduce the risk of toxicity or other adverse reactions. Since calcium and magnesium may interfere with iron absorption, upper limits of 250 and 25 mg/dose, respectively, are recommended as a part of vitamin/mineral supplements.

Some calcium supplements provide less than the recommended 600 mg of elemental calcium per tablet. It is advisable to take calcium supplements (e.g., calcium carbonate) with meals to promote absorption of the calcium.

10
Nutrition Referrals and Resources

Referral to a Registered Dietitian

To promote continuity of care, consider giving the woman a two-way referral form to carry with her (to facilitate communication between the dietitian and other caregivers). The form might include places for the primary care provider to record the purpose of the referral as well as the woman's weight, height, BMI, and hemoglobin or hematocrit and places for the dietitian to record key contents of the visit and the behavioral changes which the woman agreed to attempt to make.

What the woman can expect at the visit:

- Questions about what she eats, some of her attitudes toward food and supplements, and her daily activities (including exercise).
- Sometimes a request for some record keeping, such as 3-day food records.
- Discussion of goals for improving her nutrition.
- Some specific goals for changing behaviors—goals that are compatible with her situation and preferences.
- Written, pictorial, or taped information pertinent to the problem (e.g., an individualized eating plan, recipes, guidelines for what to do when eating out, or strategies for more comfortably meeting nutrient needs).
- Recommendations for follow-up with the dietitian or the primary care provider or both.

Eligibility for Federal Food and Nutrition Programs and Program Benefits

Program	Eligibility	Benefits
Special Supplemental Food Program for Women, Infants, and Children (WIC) Local phone number: _____-_____	Pregnant women, postpartum women (up to 6 months), breastfeeding women (up to 1 year), infants, and children (aged <5 years); must be certified to be at nutritional risk, and household income must be determined to be ≤185%[a] of the federal poverty level[b]	Individualized food packages provided monthly. These include foods such as milk, cheese, eggs, fruit juice, cereal, peanut butter or legumes, infant formula, and infant cereal Nutrition education Referrals
Commodity Supplemental Food Program (CSFP) Local phone number: _____-_____	Pregnant women, breastfeeding women, other postpartum women, infants and children (aged <6 years); household income must be determined to be ≤185%[a] of the federal poverty level	Monthly canned or packaged foods including fruits, vegetables, meats, infant formula, farina, beans, other as available
Food Stamp Program Local phone number: _____-_____	U.S. citizens, recognized refugees with visa status, and legal aliens—all from households with low income and with resources (aside from income) of ≤$2,000 (≤$3,000 with at least one elderly person[c]); eligibility is determined after formal application to local public assistance or social services agencies	Food vouchers, cards, or checks to purchase foods at participating food markets

Program	Eligibility	Benefits
Temporary Emergency Food Assistance Program (TEFAP) Local phone number: _____-_____	Households with income ≤150%[a] of the federal poverty level	Quarterly distribution: cheese, butter, rice, occasionally flour, cornmeal, and dry milk. Emergency food available once per month: dairy products, rice, flour, cornmeal
Nutrition Assistance Program (NAP) for Puerto Rico Local phone number: _____-_____	Residents of Puerto Rico who meet eligibility rules similar to those for the Food Stamp Program	Cash to be used by recipients to supplement their food budget
Food Distribution Program on Indian Reservations (FDPIR) Local phone number: _____-_____	American-Indian households living on or near reservations	Monthly canned or packaged foods, including fruits, vegetables, meats, beans, grains, flour, cereal, juice, pasta, egg mix, milk, cheese, peanut butter, honey, butter, oil, and shortening
Cooperative Extension—Expanded Food and Nutrition Education Program (EFNEP)[d] Local phone number: _____-_____	Households with children aged <19 years, with income ≤125% of the federal poverty level; at nutritional risk	Education and training on food and nutrition

Source: Adapted from Boisvert-Walsh and Kallio, with permission.[20]

[a]Some states have lower cutoff values.
[b]The federal poverty level is computed yearly. The cost of the U.S. Department of Agriculture's Thrifty Food Plan is multiplied by three and adjusted for family size and the current consumer price index.
[c]Elderly are those aged ≥60 years.
[d]EFNEP is not available in all communities.

Examples of comments or questions for the health care provider to raise at follow-up:

- Find something positive to reinforce: **It sounds like you're making a good start in increasing your energy intake to help your baby grow.**
- If no note is in the medical record, ask: **Did you meet with the dietitian after our last visit to get help with X?**
- If yes (or if there is a record of the visit): **It's good that you took the time to see the dietitian. Did you bring your referral form with you today?**
  - If the referral form has been filled out: **Tell me what you have done about X (the first behavioral change written in the plan). Do you have any questions about X? Y? Z?**
  - If there is no referral form: **What did you agree to do to accomplish X? How is it going?** Ask some specific questions related to the problem, such as: **Are you still uncomfortable after eating?**

Referral to WIC

Help low-income pregnant or postpartum women receive WIC benefits without unnecessary delay. When referring women to WIC, provide the following information: the reason for the referral; hemoglobin or hematocrit; medical risks, if any; height and weight; and special formulas required, if any, and the rationale for their use. Your local WIC agency can provide you with their standard referral forms, or you can send the information on forms of your choice or on your official stationery. Providing this information expedites the delivery of appropriate services and food packages for mothers and their infants and children. Encourage eligible pregnant and lactating women to take advantage of the information about breastfeeding and about healthful eating that WIC now provides.

Health Services Resources

The Maternal and Child Health Program (MCH), authorized under Title V, Social Security Act, resides in the Health Resources and Services Administration (HRSA) of the U.S. Department of Health and Human Services and works in partnership with state health agencies, professional groups, and providers to improve the health of mothers, children, and families.

State units of MCH and other HRSA programs promote health through standard setting and quality assurance, specialized consultation and technical assistance, inter-agency collaboration, and arrangements for direct service delivery. Nutrition services are available through each state health system as one component of comprehensive MCH care. MCH can assist you with local

---

Local Consultation and Technical Assistance

Contact your state or local department of public health for guidance or information related to maternal and child nutrition.

Local health department

_____   _____
phone number   name

State health department (Title V MCH Nutritionist)

_____   _____
phone number   name

State MCH hotline

_____
phone number

policies and referral systems for WIC, Medicaid, prenatal care access, genetic screening, perinatology centers for consultation on special conditions, therapeutic nutrition counseling, and others.

The National Center for Education in Maternal and Child Health (NCEMCH) maintains a reference collection of maternal and child health program materials; responds to information requests; provides technical assistance in educational resource development, program planning, and topical research; and provides other information services. It can also assist you in locating your state MCH representatives. NCEMCH can be reached at (703) 524-7802.

Selecting and Using Educational Materials

Materials from any source should be reviewed and evaluated before they are used in clinical practice. The following questions help to choose the best materials to use for a particular situation.

- Does the material include favorable images of the subgroups in your patient population?
- Do the visual images match the verbal message?
- Are the visual images appropriate for the age, ethnic background, and socioeconomic status of the women you serve?
- Is the information presented from a positive perspective? *(You can do it.)* Is it action oriented?
- Is the information accurate and up to date? Is it consistent with the other messages you give?
- Is the material free of subtle sales messages (e.g., if you fail at breastfeeding, there is always formula)?
- Are the recommendations practical considering the characteristics and resources of the women you serve? (For example, do they pose reasonable demands in terms of cost, time, cooking skills, and cooking and storage facilities?)

- Is written material appropriate for the reading level of the women you serve? (Consider the number of syllables in the words, the number of words in the sentences, the familiarity of key words, the type size, and the format.) Materials for low-literacy audiences should focus on the most critical patient behaviors—what to do and when to do it.
- Do the materials fit the women's stage in the change process? For example, if the women are not ready to take action, materials should not emphasize *how* to take action.

Consider the following guidelines to promote effective use of the materials selected.

- Use as few materials as possible to convey and reinforce your messages.
- Introduce the materials by briefly emphasizing the importance of the messages and giving an overview of what to expect.
- Where possible, ask for the woman's reaction to the messages. **Do you think this (the recommendation) is something that you can do?**
- Use materials to support your oral recommendations and to provide detail, such as the reasons why a particular woman should stop smoking or ways to stop.

Sources of Information About Nutritional Care During the Perinatal Period

The publications listed here are just a sampling of many useful resources. Those marked "Available from NMCHC" can be obtained from the National Maternal and Child Health Clearinghouse, 8201 Greensboro Drive, Suite 600, McLean, VA 22102 (703) 821-8955 ext. 254—usually at no cost. There is a charge for most of the other publications.

General

The following examples of manuals incorporate recommendations from the Institute of Medicine report *Nutrition During Pregnancy.*[1] They contain information to assist health care providers in the delivery of maternal nutrition services.

Alton, I., and M. Caldwell. 1990. Guidelines for Nutrition Care During Pregnancy (and revision packet). Region V, U.S. Public Health Service, U.S. Department of Health and Human Services, Chicago, IL. Available from NMCHC.

Committee for Nutrition During Pregnancy and the Postpartum Period. Asarian, J., E. Gunderson, D. Lee, V. Newman, N. Sullivan, and D. Walker. 1990. Nutrition During Pregnancy and the Postpartum Period: A Manual for Health Care Professionals. Maternal and Child Health Branch, WIC Supplemental Food Branch, California Department of Health Services, 714 P Street, Room 740, Sacramento, CA 95814. 304 pp.

Story, M., ed. 1990. Nutrition Management of the Pregnant Adolescent: A Practical Reference Guide. March of Dimes Birth Defects Foundation, White Plains, N.Y.; U.S. Department of Health and Human Services, Rockville, MD.; and U.S. Department of Agriculture, Alexandria, VA. 182 pp. Available through March of Dimes.

Examples of Prenatal Nutrition Materials Suitable for Adolescents or Young Adults

Division of Nutritional Sciences, Cornell University. 1988. A Smart Start: Nutrition for Life. Division of Nutritional Sciences, Cornell University, Ithaca, NY.

Healthy Infant Outcome Project. 1988. Hey Baby: How to Eat and Gain Right to Grow the Best Baby Possible. Regents of the University of Minnesota, Minneapolis, MN. Available from Public Health Nutrition, University of Minnesota, Box 197 Mayo Building, 420 Delaware Street, SE, Minneapolis, MN 55455.

Maternal and Infant Health. 1990. Healthy Foods, Healthy Baby. Philadelphia Department of Public Health, Philadelphia, PA. 28 pp. Available from NMCHC.

Examples of Materials for Women with Gestational Diabetes Mellitus

The first two items listed below are examples of patient education materials that are suitable for women with reading skills above the sixth grade level. The last two publications were designed for women with limited literacy skills.

ADA (American Diabetes Association). 1989. Gestational Diabetes: What to Expect. Diabetes Information Service Center, Alexandria, VA. 76 pp.

DHHS (U.S. Department of Health and Human Services). 1989. Understanding Gestational Diabetes: A Practical Guide to a Healthy Pregnancy. NIH Publ. No. 89-2788. Public Health Service, National Institutes of Health, National Institute of Child Health & Human Development, Bethesda, MD. 46 pp.

Morin, G.K., and J.O. Joynes. 1988. Healthy Eating. Diabetes Center, Inc., P.O. Box 739, Wayzata, MN 55391.

Nemanic, A., G.K. Morin, and J.O. Joynes. 1988. What Is Diabetes? Diabetes Center, Inc., P.O. Box 739, Wayzata, MN 55391.

The following publication was designed to be used by professionals in dental and other health clinics to help Navajo women with gestational diabetes control their blood sugar (and thereby decrease their susceptibility to periodontal disease). It serves as an example of a culturally sensitive teaching tool.

Pelican, S., O. Platero, G. Crawford, and D. Wise. Undated. Diabetes During Pregnancy: How to Keep the Balance. Indian Health Service Diabetes Program, 2401 Twelfth Street, NW, Albuquerque, NM 87102. 55 pp.

Information About Drugs

Berkowitz, R., D. Coustan, and T. Mochizuki. 1986. Handbook for Prescribing Medications During Pregnancy, 2nd ed. Little, Brown, and Co., Boston.

Briggs, G.F., R.K. Freeman, and S.J. Yaffe. 1990. Drugs in Pregnancy and Lactation, 3rd ed. Williams and Wilkins, Baltimore. 732 pp.

Niebyl, J.R. (ed.) 1988. Drug Use in Pregnancy, 2nd ed. Lea & Febiger, Philadelphia. 245 pp.

Information About Smoking Cessation Programs

Windsor, R.A. 1990. The Handbook to Plan, Implement and Evaluate Smoking Cessation Programs for Pregnant Women. March of Dimes Birth Defects Foundation, 1275 Mamaroneck Avenue, White Plains, NY 10605. 59 pp.

Information About Breastfeeding

The following are among many good publications for professionals.

Coates, M.-M. 1990. The Lactation Consultant's Topical Review and Bibliography of the Literature on Breastfeeding. La Leche League International, Franklin Park, IL. 188 pp. (Includes many useful citations.)

FNS (Food and Nutrition Service). 1988. Promoting Breastfeeding in WIC: A Compendium of Practical Approaches. U.S. Department of Agriculture, Alexandria, VA.

FNS (Food and Nutrition Service). 1990. WIC Breastfeeding Promotion Study and Demonstration. Phase IV Report, Volume I. U.S. Department of Agriculture, Alexandria, VA.

Jolley, S. 1990. Breastfeeding Triage Tool. Seattle-King County Department of Public Health, 110 Prefontaine Avenue South, Suite 500, Seattle, WA 98104. 94 pp.

Lawrence, R.A. 1989. Breastfeeding: A Guide for the Medical Profession, 3rd ed. C.V. Mosby, St. Louis, MO. 652 pp.

NCEMCH (National Center for Education in Maternal and Child Health). 1989. Breastfeeding: Catalog of Products from Projects Supported by the Bureau of Maternal and Child Health and Resources Development 1989. NMCHC, Washington, DC. 56 pp.

Spisak, S., and S.S. Gross. 1991. Second Followup Report: The Surgeon General's Workshop on Breastfeeding and Human Lactation. National Center for Education in Maternal and Child Health, Washington, DC. 119 pp. Available from NMCHC.

Yannicelli, S. A.E. Ernest, M.R. Neifert, and E.R.B. McCabe. 1988. Guide to Breastfeeding the Infant with PKU, 2nd ed. U.S. Department of Health and Human Services, Rockville, MD. 34 pp. Available from NMCHC.

Examples of Breastfeeding Projects to Assist Health Professionals

Best Start Breastfeeding Promotion Clearinghouse, 3500 E. Fletcher Avenue, Suite 308, Tampa, FL 33613; (800) 277-4975 or (318) 972-2119. Project Director: Carol A. Bryant, Ph.D. Offers a variety of breastfeeding promotion materials, technical assistance, and professional training materials; provides guidance on materials and program development for low literacy and minority populations.

Study Group on Human Lactation and Breastfeeding, Department of Pediatrics, University of Rochester Medical Center, 601 Elmwood Avenue, P.O. Box 777, Rochester, NY 14642; (716) 275-0088. Project Director: Ruth A. Lawrence, M.D. Provides reliable information for professionals on matters relating to human lactation and breastfeeding, including information on medications during lactation.

WellStart/San Diego Lactation Program, 4062 First Avenue, San Diego, CA 92103; (619) 295-5192. Project Director: Audrey J. Naylor, M.D., Dr. P.H. Offers a variety of educational programs for health professionals.

References

1. IOM (Institute of Medicine). 1990. Nutrition During Pregnancy. Part I, Weight Gain; Part II, Nutrient Supplements. Committee on Nutritional Status During Pregnancy and Lactation, Food and Nutrition Board. National Academy Press, Washington, DC. 468 pp.

2. IOM (Institute of Medicine). 1991. Nutrition During Lactation. Report of the Subcommittee on Nutrition During Lactation, Committee on Nutritional Status During Pregnancy and Lactation, Food and Nutrition Board. National Academy Press, Washington, DC. 309 pp.

3. Department of Health and Human Services. 1988. The Surgeon General's Report on Nutrition and Health. DHHS (PHS) Publ. No. 88-50210. Public Health Service. U.S. Government Printing Office, Washington, DC. 727 pp.

4. Department of Health and Human Services. 1990. Healthy People 2000: National Health Promotion and Disease Prevention Objectives. Public Health Service, Office of the Assistant Secretary for Health, Washington, DC. 692 pp.

5. IOM (Institute of Medicine). 1992. Nutrition Services in Perinatal Care, 2nd ed. Report of the Committee on Nutritional Status During Pregnancy and Lactation, Food and Nutrition Board. National Academy Press, Washington, DC.

6. Peoples-Sheps, M.D., W.D. Kalsbeek, E. Siegel, C. Dewees, M. Rogers, and R. Schwartz. 1991. Prenatal records: A national survey of content. Am. J. Obstet. Gynecol. 164:514-521.

7. POPRAS. 1987. Problem Oriented Perinatal Risk Assessment System; Form 1B: Physical Exam, Nutrition and Psychosocial. Comprehensive Informatics for Perinatal Health, Inc., Sacramento, CA.

8. Hollister Inc. 1986. Maternal/Newborn Record System. Hollister Inc., Libertyville, IL.

9. ACOG (American College of Obstetricians and Gynecologists). 1989. ACOG Antepartum Record. American College of Obstetricians and Gynecologists, Washington, DC.

10. Sokol, R.J., S.S. Martier, and J.W. Ager. 1989. The T-ACE questions: Practical prenatal detection of risk-drinking. Am. J. Obstet. Gynecol. 160:863-870.

11. CDC (Centers for Disease Control). 1989. CDC criteria for anemia in children and childbearing-aged women. Morbid. Mortal. Weekly Rep. 38:400-404.

12. MRC Vitamin Study Research Group. 1991. Prevention of neural tube defects: Results of the Medical Research Council Vitamin Study. Lancet 2:131-137.

13. USDA/DHHS (U.S. Department of Agriculture/U.S. Department of Health and Human Services). 1990. Nutrition and Your Health: Dietary Guidelines for Americans, 3rd ed. Home and Garden Bulletin No. 232. U.S. Department of Agriculture/U.S. Department of Health and Human Services, Washington, DC. 28 pp.

14. Anderson, S.A. (ed.) 1991. Guidelines for the Assessment and Management of Iron Deficiency in Women of Childbearing Age. Life Sciences Research Office, Federation of American Societies for Experimental Biology, Bethesda, MD. 37 pp.

15. CDC (Centers for Disease Control). 1991. Use of folic acid for prevention of spina bifida and other neural tube defects—1983-1991. Morbid. Mortal. Weekly Rep. 40:513-516.

16. Committee on Drugs, American Academy of Pediatrics. 1989. Transfer of drugs and other chemicals into human milk. Pediatrics 84:924-936.

17. Division of Nutritional Sciences, Cornell University. 1988. P. 15 in A Smart Start: Nutrition for Life. Division of Nutritional Sciences, Cornell University, Ithaca, NY.

18. Anderson, P.P., and E.S. Fenichel. 1989. Serving Culturally Diverse Families of Infants and Toddlers with Disabilities. Washington, DC: National Center for Clinical Infant Programs.

19. NRC (National Research Council). 1989. Recommended Dietary Allowances, 10th ed. Report of the Subcommittee on the Tenth Edition of the RDAs, Food and Nutrition Board, Commission on Life Sciences. National Academy Press, Washington, DC. 284 pp.

20. Boisvert-Walsh, C., and J. Kallio. 1990. Reaching out to those at highest risk. Pp. 63-84 in M. Kaufman, ed. Nutrition in Public Health. Aspen Publishers, Rockville, MD.

Index

Coventry University

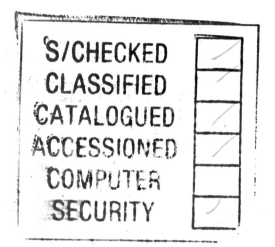